AF260546

UNTOLD
AND
RETOLD

Published in 2026 by Story Healing

ISBN number 978-1-9194803-0-5 (Paperback)

Copyright © 2026 Debra Penrice

All rights reserved. No part of this publication may be reproduced, stored in a retrieval system, or transmitted in any form or by any means, electronic or otherwise, without prior written permission from the copyright holder, except for brief excerpts used in reviews.

This is a work of fiction where some stories are based on real life experiences and retold to protect the co-authors of each story and any persons known to them. All mental well-being or health information in this book is based on the authors' professional and personal experiences, and should not be relied upon as advice or a substitute for seeking professional advice for your individual circumstances.

For my family, I grew up with your stories yet never heard enough
of them. With love

"Stories heal and stories inspire. Are you ready to share yours?"
Debs Penrice

CONTENTS

UNTOLD

AND

RETOLD

Foreword

Adam Brooks

When I first sat down to write my story for *Untold and Retold*, I didn't realise I was opening a door that would change how I saw myself and how I understood healing. What began as a chapter soon became a mirror. I'd thought I was simply contributing a story, one among many. But in truth, I was unblocking something buried deep within me: a version of myself I'd been waiting to meet for years. That's the thing about storytelling, you think you're writing about your past, but really, you're writing your way back to your truth. I've always believed that people's stories matter, that they can heal, connect, and give language to the parts of life we often carry in silence. But I hadn't realised the depth of that truth until I began to tell my own. From starting to write a chapter with a mixture of curiosity and caution, the journey that unfolded surprised me. It's one thing to coach others to 'open up' or to guide people through their journey of understanding; it's another to sit with your own words and accept you're still learning, still healing, still growing.

Debs' vision for this book with the phrase 'unblocking the hidden stories that shape our lives' resonated deeply with me. Because that's what it feels like when you begin to put words to the things you've long kept hidden. At first, it's uncomfortable... confronting, even. You start by writing what you think people will understand, only to realise you're really writing what you need to understand. You think you're telling the story of what happened, but in the process, you find meaning in how it changed you.

Untold and Retold is a collection of stories and a live conversation between human beings who have chosen courage over comfort. Each chapter, each reflection, holds a moment where someone decided that silence was no longer serving them. These stories offer an invitation to recognise how healing begins when we stop trying to hold everything so tightly. There's a rhythm that runs through every chapter of this book, a rhythm of rediscovery. As I read these stories, I saw pieces of my own journey reflected back at me. I recognised the silence that sits beneath unspoken pain. I recognised the tension between who we are and who we think we're meant to be. And I recognised the moment when you realise that healing doesn't come from fixing the past, but from finally listening to it.

That's what this book does so beautifully, it listens. It listens to the woman rediscovering herself after heartbreak, to the man learning to speak after years of silence, to the quiet strength of someone who has carried grief yet still chooses to love. It listens without judgement, without expectation, with a kind of openness that reminds you that being human is messy, imperfect, and magnificent all at once. Debs has created something extraordinary here. Not just a collection of writing, but a space, a sacred space, where stories can breathe. She gathered people from different walks of life, each bringing their own craft, experience, and vulnerability. Therapists, coaches, healers, all connected by a shared understanding that healing isn't linear. There's no one-size-fits-all solution, no single method or quick fix. Healing is a journey made up of learning, moving, growing, connecting, understanding, respecting, and revealing, all the words that title these chapters, but also, all the stages of what it means to live a human life.

As I wrote more, I found myself reflecting on the men in my life, the generations before me, the ones who taught me what love looked like even when they didn't know how to show it. I realised how many stories we inherit without question. Stories about strength, masculinity, love, failure, and success. Stories that tell us how to behave, how to feel, what to hide. And sometimes, it's not until we sit down to write that we notice those inherited narratives still shaping how we live. Writing gave me the distance to see those patterns clearly and the courage to change them. In the chapters, I see echoes of that same transformation. Gerwyn's story of pain and connection in 'Revealing' speaks to the quiet bravery it takes for men to share their emotional truth. Each of these voices contributes a different kind of medicine.

Whether you dip into one chapter at a time and reflect on how it relates to your own experiences, or whether you read the whole book, I hope these stories inspire you to consider the power of your own stories. Em's 'Honouring' chapter brings us back to the heart of it all, that stories are how we remember, how we honour, and how we pass on love.

For me, it was all about love, or perhaps more accurately, learning what love really is, and what it isn't. My story started as a chapter, but as the words began to flow, together with editorial support, I realised it was just the first layer of something much bigger. That's the power of this process: when we give ourselves permission to speak honestly, we don't just release the pain, we begin to rewrite the way we see ourselves. What strikes me most about this collection is how universal these moments are. You don't have to be a writer, a therapist, or a coach to relate to them. You just have to be human. Because every one of us has an untold story that wants to be heard, or one that needs to be reframed through compassion instead of pain.

That's what storytelling does. It allows us to revisit our memories without reliving them. It turns our past into wisdom. It takes something that once hurt and turns it into something that can help someone else. There's a sacred exchange that happens when one person shares their story and another person sees themselves within it. That's where healing begins, in the space between storyteller and listener. While continuing my own writing journey, I carry the lessons of *Untold and Retold* with me. This collaboration reminded me that healing isn't something we do alone. We heal in community. We heal through witnessing one another's truths. We heal through words spoken, written, whispered, or even held silently in our hearts until we're ready to release them.

So, as you turn the page and step into these stories, I invite you to do one thing: slow down. Let each chapter meet you where you are. Notice what stirs, what resonates, what stays with you after you close the book. Because maybe, just maybe, there's a part of your own story that's ready to be told or retold in a new way.

And if there is, I hope this book gives you the courage to begin.

Adam

Adam Brooks is a business coach, writer, and speaker based in South Wales. He specialises in human-centred leadership and personal growth, helping people and organisations reconnect with their purpose, values, and emotional truth. His work explores how vulnerability, curiosity, and conversation lead to deeper connection and more meaningful success in business and in life.

PREFACE

Debs Penrice

Have you ever had one of those conversations, where, for some reason you're excited, and afterwards, you remember every word? That's the vibration of the words... rooted in love or emotion. Words resonate more strongly when they trigger our emotions. But we often interpret those emotions by attaching stories to them or our memory recalls other related stories, associated with those emotions or words.

Stories can teach, connect, inspire, harm or heal. But what about the inner stories that remain unspoken? Or the stories that get re-told over and over until they make an impact?

The energy behind stories is powerful. Throughout history, stories have been the foundation of our existence and connection. They help us remember experiences, build relationships and develop our identities. They help heal us and they inspire us to change. This book was created to honour those hidden moments of reckoning, reflection and renewal.

Far too many of us reach a point in life when we reflect on what we've lived through and the choices we've made, wondering what we might want to do with the time still ahead of us. For some, it hits hard after a life-changing event. Perhaps a loss, a change in health, or a quiet realisation that now is the time to do something meaningful. For others, that reflection happens when work finally slows down and we are ready for retirement.

Gathering a team of authors together to write this book was an obvious move for me because there's no singular, defined path for healing: I wanted this book to explore the many ways that stories heal. Healing can happen by building a puzzle of hundreds of pieces of self-awareness, joining up approaches to nurture your body or relax your mind. In curating this book, I met talented coaches, therapists and healers, all making significant transformations with their work. Each offers a piece of the puzzle from their own path or from a successful client relationship.

You might see a part of yourself in these pages. Maybe one chapter will resonate especially for you? All our short stories are designed to give you hope. Perhaps a story will stir a memory, offer comfort, or spark the idea that you, too, have something worth sharing. Because you do.

Debs Penrice

Introduction

If you're part way through life and feeling you want greater fulfilment, or you're looking back at a long career and rediscovering your passions, or simply wondering what might be your next level of success, then this book is for you. It contains short stories that invite you to think about how ordinary life experiences can lead to transformation and healing.

It's never too late to explore your story. Writing is a sacred, creative art that connects our mind, heart and gut instincts. And if you feel the nudge to write it, speak it, or shape your stories into something more, I hope this book shows you how powerful that can be.

To support you, I'd encourage you to go on a journey of self-awareness that will help you to get to know all the things that drive your creativity and bring you joy. Since studying psychology in my counselling and hypnotherapy courses, I have learned how anxiety cannot co-exist with creativity. Anxiety and fear stop us being creative. But the good news is, if we take action to be creative, peace reigns and anxiety is forced to retreat.

There are curious and joyful elements in all kinds of creative arts. In *Living the Artist's Way*, Julia Cameron writes about four essential tools for encouraging creativity: morning pages, artist dates, walking and writing for guidance.

I've been following my intuitive guidance for over three years since a foundation course with Chris Stanley, one of the co-authors of this book. That guidance led me to re-train as a therapist and create this collaborative piece.

To help you navigate our stories – each chapter is a stand-alone short story – I want to share a few key concepts that we, as co-authors, were all aware of as we wrote.

Maslow's hierarchy of needs

This is a psychological model that describes human motivation as a series of levels, often shown as a pyramid. Maslow believed that people must generally satisfy more basic needs before focusing on the higher-level ones.

- Physiological needs: At the bottom of the pyramid are the essentials for our survival – food, water, rest, shelter and other physical requirements. Without these, little else matters.
- Safety needs: Once survival is secured, people seek stability and protection. This includes physical safety, health, secure housing, financial stability and freedom from danger.
- Love and belonging: We are wired to naturally crave connection. Once our physiological and safety needs are met, relationships, friendships, family bonds, and a sense of community become our focus.
- Esteem needs: Next, we strive for recognition and self-respect, including growing our confidence, achievement and the feeling of being valued by others.
- Self-actualisation: At the top of the hierarchy is the drive to fulfil our potential, creating purpose and meaning in life. This can mean creativity, personal growth, pursuing passions or living in alignment with deeper values.

Why sleep matters

Sleep isn't just resting; it's your body's way of fixing, sorting, cleaning and learning. Imagine sleep with a team of night-shift workers who come out when you close your eyes. They tidy up, repair what's broken and get you ready for a brand-new day.

- Your body heals: Muscles repair, cuts and scrapes heal faster, and your immune system (your body's guard against germs) gets stronger.
- Your brain processes: All the busy thinking from the day makes "mess" in your brain, and sleep cleanses that away like a night-time cleaning crew.
- You learn better: Things you studied or practiced during the day get sorted and stored, like putting books neatly on the right shelf in a library.

About 20% of your sleep cycle is rapid eye movement (REM) sleep – the parts of the night when you dream. Think of it like your brain's movie theatre. But it's not just for fun – it has the very important job of emptying your so-called stress bucket.

Every day, worries and frustrations drop into your stress bucket. If the bucket gets too full, you feel grumpy or overwhelmed. REM sleep empties the bucket by replaying tricky feelings in a safe way. It's almost like your brain is saying, "It's okay, we can handle this now."

Boosting creativity: REM also helps you connect new ideas, like when you suddenly solve a problem or come up with a clever thought. So, sleep is not "lost time". It's the most important superhero power you have. Without it, you may struggle with anxiety, you can't learn as well, and your stress bucket starts to overflow.

Your brain's rational versus emotional responses

Your brain is complex and yet, if we simplify our understanding of it, there are two parts to understand better:

- The intellectual-thinking brain (prefrontal cortex) is the smart part at the very front of your head. It helps you make plans, solve problems and think rationally before you act. It's like the wise boss inside your brain.
- The emotional-feeling brain includes the primitive parts of your brain that help you notice danger, emotions and feelings. It

reacts fast, before your thinking brain has time to catch up. It's like your brain's safety officer or alarm system.

When something in your environment triggers your brain to suspect you're in danger, your thinking moves instantly into the emotional brain because it's much quicker to respond. Then your body might do one of four things:

- Fight – anger rises to get ready to argue, shout or push back.
- Flight – adrenaline rises to run away or try to escape.
- Freeze – stop moving, like a deer standing still in headlights.
- Fawn – please others so the danger goes away, like saying, "Okay, okay, I'll do whatever you want."

This happens in your sympathetic nervous system, which is like a network of super-fast wires carrying messages all through your body. But another system, the parasympathetic nervous system, helps calm you back down after danger, like pressing the "relax" button. So, your brain has a boss part (thinking) and an alarm part (feeling), and sometimes the alarm part takes over. But when we learn to relax more, your boss brain can help you make good choices and stick to your long-term goals.

Motivating flows of neurotransmitters

Your brain makes special chemicals that act like messengers. They tell your body how to feel. Some make you happy and connected, others warn you about danger. These motivating neurotransmitters include:

- Serotonin, the "sunshine" chemical, which helps you feel calm, safe, and steady.
- Dopamine, the "reward" chemical, gives you a burst of excitement when you get something good or achieve a goal.
- Oxytocin, the "hug" chemical, makes you feel close to people you trust and love.

These are like your happy helpers. Dopamine is wonderful in small doses, like when you finish a puzzle, score a goal or get a high-five. But here's the tricky part: if your dopamine level shoots up high (from eating too much sugar, playing video games for hours or taking harmful drugs), it can come crashing down afterward and some of the receptors close from the overload. That crash makes your brain think, *I want that big high again!'* but because some receptors have closed, it takes even more dopamine to reach the same level. This creates a loop that can grow into addiction, as your brain keeps chasing the high but never feels satisfied for long. It's like going on a rollercoaster that shoots you up super high and then drops you fast — fun at first but exhausting if you ride it over and over.

Sometimes, your brain sends out warning chemicals:

- Adrenaline and norepinephrine give you a quick jolt of energy to run or fight if you're in danger.
- Cortisol, the "stress chemical," keeps you on high alert if trouble lasts a while.

These are important chemicals when you *really* need them, but if they hang around too long, they make you feel worn out and anxious. The best way to keep your brain's feel-good chemicals balanced is through natural actions: sleep, exercise, laughter, hugs, learning new skills and spending time with people you love. They keep the happy helpers steady and strong, without the crash.

Perspective and focus – our reticular activating system

Inside your brain, there's a tiny switchboard called the reticular activating system (RAS). Its job is to notice what's important to you and shine a spotlight on it. Imagine you want a green car, or you just got new red shoes. Suddenly, you start spotting red shoes everywhere! Did the world suddenly fill up with red shoes? No. You and your brain decided, *'Green cars or red shoes matter now,'* so it notices and points them out. It feels like we attract more of something, but really, our powerful RAS is just showing us what was already there or is possible for us to achieve. It's like when you highlight words in a book — the words don't appear out of nowhere, but they stand out because you marked them.

RAS is important because, if you focus on good things (like kindness, fun, or opportunities to learn), your brain will notice more of them. If you focus on worries or problems, your brain will keep pointing those out instead. So, the secret power is what you pay attention to grows bigger in your mind. Your RAS is like your brain's filter to help you see and achieve more of what you're looking for.

Hopefully these concepts help you become more self-aware as you navigate our stories. At the end of each chapter, there are questions for you to reflect on, if you'd like.

My co-authors have shared a fraction of their stories, and you can find out more about them by following their QR codes in the author biographies at the end. Maybe it's time to unblock your soul story too?

1

LEARNING

Lisa Williams Edgar

Stories help us learn. We read with our children from their earliest days, sharing picture books or making up stories to excite their imaginations. But these stories have a purpose – they teach our children about the world. The earliest stories we share with children are often about kindness or emotions and relationships, or about different places and the animal kingdom. Then they grow into learning about risk and conflict through stories about super heroes, adversity and even crime or mystery. *The Famous Five* and *Nancy Drew* mysteries have made way for a plethora of more modern stories, such as Robin Stevens's *Murder Most Unladylike* series.

In adulthood, stories continue to play a key role in learning. In education, we share case studies of real people and scenarios, and in business and science, we create story narratives to explain data or new concepts. We use metaphor to simplify stories and to help the brain understand what is possible or the change it needs to make. Metaphors can help our brains to relax by taking a common concept and helping the subconscious to process its deeper meaning. The mind can choose which parts of the metaphor resonate most with our personal experience.

When I first met Lisa on my journey to retrain as a solution focused hypnotherapist, she was regularly writing new metaphors for her clients and her trainees. One of my favourite metaphors is the one Lisa shares here, which I now use with clients who are seeking to develop more flexible thinking.

The Little Pebble

There once was a lively stream that flowed through a serene valley before joining the river below. Within the stream were many pebbles, each unique in size and shape. Among these, a small smooth pebble stood out for its ability to glide effortlessly with the water's current. It bounced, tumbled and rolled, experiencing the stream from various angles and perspectives, enjoying the journey with ease and curiosity.

Not far from this pebble lay a larger, grey, more rigid stone, firmly settled in the streambed. It had been there for years, steadfast and unyielding, watching the small pebble's adventures with a mix of admiration and apprehension. The large stone wondered how the pebble could so freely embrace the changing current; how it could find joy in the unpredictable flow of the water.

One day, the larger stone asked the pebble, "How do you manage to explore and enjoy the stream so freely? How do you adapt to the ever-changing waters?"

The small pebble replied, "I embrace the flow, let go of the need to remain still. It's in the movement that I find new views and exciting new experiences."

Inspired by the pebble's words, the larger stone decided to let go, to allow the stream's current to gently shift its position. As it did so, it started to see the valley from new angles, to experience aspects of the stream it had never noticed before. The larger stone realised that its strength and stability weren't just in staying put; they were also in its ability to adapt and move with the water.

As the stone became more flexible in its approach, it discovered that what it once saw as the limits of its world were merely boundaries it had set for itself. Now, moving slightly with the stream, it saw beyond its usual spot – glimpses of the surrounding landscape, the dance of light on the water's surface that created a mosaic of colours and patterns.

The large stone now finds joy in this new way of experiencing the world. It has realised that it can embrace change while maintaining its own essence. It has learned to recall pleasant memories and images from this new perspective, enriching its existence within the stream.

Lisa Williams-Edgar: www.newhorizontraining.co.uk

UNBLOCKING YOUR HIDDEN STORIES:

What are your thoughts after reading this metaphor?

Which stories from your childhood have shaped your thinking?

2

MOVING

Becky Clark

Stories help us move through our emotions. When we witness a character in a book taking on a challenge or enduring a traumatic experience, our natural empathy kicks in. By hearing their story, we give ourselves space to release some of our own stories and feelings too. The space to acknowledge and process events without the pressure to relive our own version of events is a wonderful gift because our brains can't tell the difference between imagined and real thoughts. If you bring a memory to mind right now, you'll feel a shadow of the original emotions. So, some stories are best told through drama performance, dance and movement.

I first met Becky when I joined a Thrive networking event at her jointly-owned wellness centre, Goldney House. She told me, "Learning to move sober was one of the rawest, most powerful things I've ever done. It felt awkward at first, even shameful. But it was the gateway to power. Dancing, shaking, expressing without apology – that's how I say to the world: I trust myself more than I need your approval." Becky's Somatic Disco isn't just an event. It's a reclamation. It's a homecoming. It's where she creates, embodies, leads and celebrates what she calls "the light that was always mine to carry."

Her story is one that might be scarily familiar to many young people who are still learning how to process their emotions and who continue to feel disconnected. Yet sometimes, the story remains untold and the truth passes through the body, no longer harmful once the motion takes over and dissipates the emotion. Not all stories need words.

Where am I?

It's dark. I can hear the low hum and vibration of the bass rhythm thudding beneath me through the concrete floor. I hear the chaotic chatter of people shouting and moving around, the thud of feet past my face, shuffling and scurrying. The ground beneath my numb cheekbone is cold and hard. As I slowly pry open one eye, sparks of light shoot across my vision like lasers, chaotic and disorienting.

Where am I?

Before I can make sense of the scene, a tidal wave of excruciating pain crashes through my whole being. It's not isolated to one part of my body; rather, it saturates my every cell, my every fibre. Even through the haze of my drug cocktail and sleepless nights, the pain is unmistakable, sharp, raw and intolerable. I suppose this is what dying feels like – a slow, agonising descent into helplessness. A shadow self in a black hole leaving the earth. As I weave in and out of consciousness, I make out a blur of feet surrounding me. A familiar face leans down.

"Bex, Bex, can you hear me?"

I recognise the voice, a thread of connection anchoring me to reality. Relief briefly flickers in my chest – I'm not completely alone. Before I can form another thought, I sense my body being lifted, but I feel distant, like I'm trapped inside a heavy leaden shell. My body is on some moving but hard unyielding surface. I glimpse daylight ahead, but it's a dull, distant promise. The excruciating pain of the movement jolts me back into semi-consciousness as I am carried through the darkness into a grey, desolate world, to a derelict car park – and then everything goes black once again.

When I open my eyes, a woman in blue hovers beside me, her voice soft yet direct. She asks my name and the date, but all I can say is, "Ouchhh."

My body feels broken, shattered. Any movement sends fresh knives of pain slicing through me. I hear the word 'roundabout' and realise I'm being transported in an ambulance, thrown around violently with each turn.

"Pain," I say. It's the only word I can form.

They search for a vein, desperate to find a way to give me relief, but dehydration has closed off the pathways. "We'll have to give Oromorph orally," the medic tells me. The cruel twist – no instant relief. Only the waiting. The grinding, gnawing agony.

As the ambulance lurches on, my mind drifts to my mother. I can almost feel her hand holding mine, even though I know she isn't there. Shame, fear and confusion rise up, heavier than the pain – shame about how far I have fallen, about the choices that have led me here. I wonder what she would think of me now – bruised, broken, barely alive and the heart ache the future may hold for her.

I am 24 years old. Lying here, I realise I have spent most of my life searching outside of myself – for approval, validation, belonging. Performing, pleasing, numbing. Always numbing. Through drugs, through alcohol, and silently, insidiously, through food.

Where am I?

I squint and my face warms as the bright sun kisses my skin. It smells like a glorious afternoon at Slimbridge. As I sit in my wheelchair, pondering and staring out onto the lake with its flock of geese, I am grateful to my mum for taking me out on a day trip. It can get lonely on my own, stuck up in my bedroom. Two ducks have gathered at my feet, interested in the loaf of bread, most of which I seem to have inhaled while cloud watching, not even noticing it going in my mouth. I feel bloated and thirsty. I'm familiar with this feeling, for sure. It's not just the loaf of bread; it's the six-pack of Twix I secretly binged first thing this morning. How could I not when I woke up thinking about them? It was that usual niggling thought of how I'd chucked them in the bin the night before, still in their wrappers. The niggle turned into a compulsion until I fished them out of the bin and gorged on them. It's a mysterious game that I often shame myself with; me and my trusty secret companion – food. Eating is my safe place and it never judges me.

Where am I?

As I stand in line, the two ladies in front of me cheer and clap together. I feel flushed and hot, and a sudden state of panic creeps in as I realise that I'm next into the hot seat. *Aghhh...* it's a hard act to follow as she's getting cheered for her efforts over the previous week. I feel the clamminess of my hand as I give my book to and make eye contact with the woman in charge. She looks at me with kind, anticipating eyes as I step towards the scales with a nervy, awkward shuffle. I'm the youngest one here, so I often feel the maternal energy in the room. I'm nearly 16, and they know how much I need this. They know that my life will be so much better once I've lost this extra weight. So, they kindly turn a blind eye. I'm here with my mum. We come as a pair. In fact, I look forward to this meeting every week because mum and I celebrate afterwards with fish and chips, no matter what the scales say. The evening is filled with love and connection. As I slip my shoes off, I feel a mixture of emotions. I've avoided fluids all afternoon in a bid to weigh less. But that often gives me a headache, so I'm excited that I'll be able to rehydrate soon. But I also feel a little twitchy, remembering that I got caught out four days ago and had to buy a shop sandwich at school. The shame starts to creep in, but I bat it away with a deep breath as I step on...

Where am I?

My friends glide ahead of me, light on their feet, all limbs and laughter – lean, pretty, effortless. They move with the kind of ease that makes walking, and maybe even life, look weightless. It's the tidy rhythm of succeeding at life. I, meanwhile, pant up the hill, dragging my legs like they're filled with wet sand. Each step lands with a thud, my breath catching somewhere between my chest and throat. There's a rhythm to my body too – but my rhythm is slow, reluctant, heavy. I'm not sure if this heaviness I feel as I continue to pant up the hill is physical or internal. Either way, it forces a memory into the forefront of my mind.

My 9-year-old self, feeling unworthy, ashamed, left behind, rejected and incapable, dreaming of a delivery of a bottle of Sunny Delight and family-sized bag of McCoy crisps, to sooth her emotions. A yummy tasty satisfying memory all wrapped up in her favourite film of all time *The Sound of Music*. And the best bit of all – time spent with Mum, the greatest love/hate addiction of all time. She longs to be with her yet is irritated and frustrated by her; Mum is her everything.

The path feels longer beneath me, steeper somehow, as if it knows I'm carrying more than just the weight of my body. My skin prickles, not from exertion alone, but from the dull ache of not quite belonging. My friends chat ahead, their voices drifting back to me like music from a distant room. I force myself along, trying to keep up, trying not to let the heaviness inside me show. As I straggle behind, I walk under a mirrored underpass. I am stopped in my tracks with disgust as I take in the girl standing in front of me. Is this actually me? I want to claw at my own reflection, feeling like an outsider in my own skin. I reach down to my tummy and pinch my fat, making myself wince. This quiet cruelty and private self-punishment are easy to do secretly, without anyone noticing; a sharp reminder of the shame and self-hate that have become my make-up.

My friends don't see it; don't see me. They laugh and move as one. But I always feel just a beat behind, slightly out of sync. I wonder what they really think when they glance back at me, red-faced and silent. The paranoia hums quietly beneath everything else – maybe they notice, maybe they don't, but either way, I know I'm different. Maybe there's a place where I'd fit in more easily, a group whose rhythm mirrors mine. Or maybe I'm just not built for blending in. Maybe I was never meant to move with the usual flow.

Where am I?

I sit on the rooftop terrace of my beautiful wellness centre, the warm sun kissing my skin. I feel a wave of safety and knowing wash over me, prompting an expansive, deep sigh. I'm finalizing the content for my new signature Flip Formula. It's a method to help others shake and move stagnant energy out of the body while rewiring their self-belief and dissolving shame blocks. I start to reflect and turn inward...

I once again connect into my body, trusting this process now like an old friend. A feeling arises. A thought. One that brings me face-to-face with the little lost Becky that I was. I lock in deeper and meet her with heartfelt eyes.

Heavy with compassion for the girl who once thought she was broken. I offer her kindness. I offer her reassurance. I remind her that her body was never the problem. It was always the path home.

If only she had known that freedom, joy and wholeness were waiting on the other side of shame and survival. On the other side of the numbing.

That the answer wasn't out there – it was within. To feel. To move. To listen. To build an internal empire rooted in safety and trust.

That there was always a place where she belonged. A place where she could be accepted in every capacity, with unconditional love. A place where she ruled and was queen. A place where she could play, be real, be whole and electric. I tell her now that there was a reason for all of it.

A bigger purpose behind the pain.

A deeper meaning behind the missteps.

Because the movement is finally here...

It's arrived...

It's gathering momentum...

It's going to be bigger than she ever imagined...

And well worth the wait…
For she now has the rhythm that she used to run from.

Becky Clark: www.beckyclarkcoaching.com

UNBLOCKING YOUR HIDDEN STORIES:

What comes up for you after reading this story?

What might move you in a different direction for the future?

3

GROWING

Tor Obermaier

Growing from childhood into adulthood we hear many more stories and experience our own moments of connection and life events. As we explored in the last chapter, the stories we carry live not just in our minds, but in our bodies. Over the years, they can settle into us as tension, aches, fatigue or even a quiet heaviness we can't quite name. When I joined Tor's Nia Dance Retreat in a beautiful location in the Forest of Dean, I found out firsthand how dance can help you grow and lift your mood. As Tor says, "One of the most powerful ways I've found to release those stories is through movement – letting the body speak when words aren't enough. That discovery is what first drew me to Nia, and it's what continues to transform both me and the women I dance with. I've always loved the ebb and flow of the seasons which move and change in ways that can reflect the movement our bodies need. I am fortunate to live nestled between the Forest of Dean and the Wye Valley, where we get the different seasons in all their glory! The vibrant colours of early summer and the glistening of the River Wye which looks gorgeous from a distance. Then they give way to late summer and the colours deepen, through to the array of shades of autumn and the stillness of winter. I love them all and how they guide our own energy levels."

The first Nia dance routine that Tor learned and then taught her class was called Bloom. As she led her classes through this routine from week to week, she noticed the women blossoming. In this story, Tor recounts a story from one of her first dance groups. "One lady, who I would describe as now in full bloom, decided to unleash herself into this transformative journey. This is her story, and I hope her awakening encourages you as much as it did me."

From seed to full bloom

Standing at the front of the dance studio, mirrors reflecting the faces of my new students, I felt a tingle of nervous anticipation. I'd carefully chosen the end of August to begin my Nia classes – it's always felt like a time of fresh starts. As a former schoolteacher, this time of year brought that familiar back-to-school energy: new classes, new relationships, new beginnings.

As I've grown older, I've tried to line up more with the rhythms of nature. I'm officially a winterer now – someone who deliberately slows down with the season and conserves energy, just like the natural world around me.

Starting those first Nia classes felt like a bold new chapter. Dance had always been part of my life – making up routines to ABBA in the living room, jumping off benches to *Fame* at school discos, raving through the nineties. My three daughters still say some of their favourite memories are of the whole family dancing in the garden after dinner. Dance gives me freedom: to feel, to express, to connect. But even with that lifelong love, my mind still buzzed with questions. Would the women enjoy it? Could I guide them clearly? Would it feel chaotic or connected? Imposter syndrome was very much on patrol.

Beth walked in just before we started and introduced herself.

"I love to dance," she said, "but I haven't really moved my body in a long time."

Great, I thought. *She's going to love this.*

Seed

Once the class began, I noticed Beth's face didn't quite match the joy I was expecting. She frowned, sighed and even stamped her foot at times. It left me a bit rattled – this was my first class, after all, and

I wanted everyone to enjoy it. Afterwards, she came straight up to me.

"Why didn't you stop and teach the moves?" she asked. "I didn't know what I was doing." Her frustration was palpable.

I paused, then said gently, "You know, Beth, part of the joy of Nia is letting go. It's not about getting every move 'right.' It's about allowing the music to move through you, and seeing what your body wants to do in that moment."

She hesitated. "I suppose I've just grown up with this expectation that things have to be done right. My dad was a rugby player – he believed in practising until you perfect it. Maybe I do need to let go a bit... though that feels scary. But maybe I don't have to get every move right."

A seed had been planted that day. Comparison is a thief. We idolise qualities we think we should have and then feel like failures when we fall short. For many women, walking into a room full of strangers – each with different bodies, stories, strengths – is daunting. But given the right environment, they all have the capacity to bloom.

Bud

To my surprise – and joy – Beth came back the next week. She had signed up for six sessions and, as I quickly learned, when this woman commits, she commits wholeheartedly.

Week by week, I watched her let go a little more. Yes, she still got frustrated when she 'made a mistake,' but it didn't stop her showing up. I'll never forget the delight on her face when she realised she could bend over and touch the floor.

"I haven't been able to do that in years!" she exclaimed.

It was a breakthrough – not just in her flexibility, but in her trust that this movement was doing something real and good for her body.

And the laughter! My mum comes to one of my Nia classes, and there's one movement that makes her howl every time. She literally cries with laughter as she dances. It's contagious and beautiful and utterly freeing. There's no better therapy.

Flower

In a short space of time, Nia became non-negotiable for Beth. It was her time – her rock. And with every class, her movements grew freer and more expressive.

Two months after her first class, she came to a Nia day retreat. I watched from the stage as she danced the Bloom routine, radiating happiness. During the day, she shared something deeply personal: she was on a journey to discover who she really was, underneath the people-pleaser she'd become. She said she'd spent her life attending to everyone else's needs and had lost sight of herself.

Nearly every woman in the room nodded in recognition. It's a story as old as time. So many of us have lost ourselves in patriarchy – trained to shrink, to be polite, to stay quiet. To keep the peace. But when I saw Beth dance that day, she looked anything but diminished. Her movements were fluid and uninhibited. She was herself.

Full bloom

Over the weeks, Beth truly bloomed. In class, we now joke about "embodying our inner Beth" – going all in, no holding back. She jumps, glides, skips, melts. She lets herself rest. At the end of class, when I say, "We're going to the floor," she's there before I even finish the sentence.

Her body moves freely now – no choreography, no pressure, just presence. No more frustrated stamping (unless that's what her body wants to do!). Her body shape has changed too. And the most powerful shift of all?

On one retreat day, Beth shared that she'd been on antidepressants for years.

"I haven't taken any medication for three months," she told the group. "I've finally given myself permission to be me. I've realised I've been suppressing my emotions for years, and that makes me feel sad. But when I dance, I feel so free. I feel lighter."

There wasn't a dry eye in the room.

At the end of a recent class, as we gathered for our usual circle hug (we all love a good cwtch in Nia!), Beth said, "You know, when I first came to Nia, I never imagined I'd find such a beautiful community of women where I feel totally free to be myself."

That was exactly what I'd always hoped to create. A space where women can come home to themselves. Nia has given us that—freedom to move, to express, to heal, and, most of all, to let go.

Tor Obermaier: www.tor-obermaier.live.baluu.io

UNBLOCKING YOUR HIDDEN STORIES:

What comes up for you after reading this story - where have you blossomed?

If there's more growing to do, which direction might you like to go in?

4

CONNECTING

Chris Stanley

Before we were writing, families passed down their histories by telling stories round the campfire, at mealtimes and at other moments of gathering. Still now, parents and families swap daily stories and anecdotes over dinner, in homes where that ritual has survived. Stories matter because they're one of our oldest forms of connection. Only by listening to a person's stories can we really get to know them. We begin to understand their perspective and feel empathy for them. As we hear their joys and struggles, we can relate better and build meaningful connections. Whether the connection is familial, a friendship, or a more remote acquaintance, the bond will strengthen through genuine listening and open story-sharing. Stories help us to identify common ground and deepen our bonds. New connections become friends when they meet for a coffee and share a story or two. It doesn't matter how brief or deep the story, it creates a spark of connection – words have power. The sounds our voices make to create words vibrate with energy and everything we say or hear transfers that energy into emotions within our bodies. Higher vibration energies come from joyful stories, while lower vibration words carry a heaviness that passes those emotions on and the need for healing may result.

I first met Chris at a business training event. We swapped notes about how we can all feel the energy change in a room when someone speaks with joy or with negative emotions in their voices. As Chris shared more about his own spiritual path, I knew I wanted to learn from him.

The connections we make on the earthly plane and the ones that are possible in the energy or spirit world are becoming more widely accepted, as we cross over into the world of science and quantum physics and mechanics. In this story, Chris shares how his spiritual journey unfolded.

Already on the path

It began on a cool quiet Tuesday evening that held the weight of early autumn. It was the evening that everything changed. I had just made a cup of tea when the message came through from Mia. She was someone I'd known in passing – warm smile, a voice that always made you feel like you'd been heard. She mentioned the spiritual circle she was running and said she felt I might be a good fit. But before confirming anything, she asked if we could have a quick phone chat.

"It's important to know if this space is the right fit," she explained.

The call wasn't formal or pressured, but it carried a sense of intentionality. It was more than a casual invite – it was a conversation about alignment. She wanted to hear where I was on my journey, what I was seeking, and whether the group would be able to support that. It didn't feel like an interview in the traditional sense, but it did invite honesty. And I appreciated that. We talked openly, and something in her energy made me feel instantly at ease.

By the end of the call, she said warmly, "I'd love for you to join us. We meet every Tuesday evening. Come if it feels right."

My spiritual journey hadn't been linear. I had attended several open circles already, but none felt quite right for me. I'd dabbled in meditation, felt pulled by energy in rooms, and had unexplainable dreams that stayed with me for years. But I'd never felt fully seen in any of them. That night, I said yes without hesitation.

Tuesday: The arrival

I arrived early for the first session. Mia had given me an address that led to a row of terraced houses, their front doors opening directly onto the pavement. The kind of street where every doorstep had seen countless comings and goings – brickwork weathered but full of character. At first glance, each house looked similar, but small personal touches set them apart – a pot of herbs here, a brightly painted door there, wind chimes, children's art in the windows.

Hers was easy to spot. Soft golden light spilled from the downstairs window, the faint sound of instrumental music weaving into the evening air. I stood for a moment on the quiet street, gathering myself before knocking. Mia smiled when she saw me and wrapped me in a great big hug. Her energy was out of this world. I felt it immediately – grounding yet uplifting, soft but powerful.

"Welcome," she said warmly. In that moment, I knew I was exactly where I was meant to be.

Inside, the room breathed. It wasn't just warm – it was sacred. Candles flickered on a central table, surrounded by a circle of mismatched chairs casually scattered with cushions and draped in soft blankets. Shelves overflowed with books and crystals. The scent of sandalwood and lavender mingled in the air. It felt lived-in. Held. Real.

That first night, Mia explained the ground rules: what's shared in the room stays in the room. It was an unspoken kind of confidentiality, reinforced by quiet nods and mutual respect. She spoke of intuition and Spirit. Of signs. Of memories. Of the things we'd hidden or dismissed.

I shared a memory from when I was two years old, nearly three. A memory of confidently telling my parents that there was a duck pond around a corner. I'd never seen it; I just knew it was there. And there was a pond. The group listened – not with disbelief, but with understanding. I felt myself exhale. For the first time in a long time, I felt... recognised.

As the evening drew to a close, Mia invited us to pull an oracle card from a small deck on the side. We each took a turn, holding our cards gently before reading their messages aloud, if we wanted to. Some shared. Some simply smiled and nodded, keeping the message close to their chests.

Mine read:

You are already on the path. Trust it.

A lump rose in my throat.

Shortly afterwards, we closed the circle with a brief grounding, as Mia gently guided us back into our bodies. Then came the soft hum of casual conversation, people putting on coats, sharing quiet goodbyes, and hugging as if they'd known each other for years. A couple lingered to chat with Mia, and I found myself hanging back too, reluctant to leave the cocoon of safety that had been woven. Eventually, I stepped out into the night. The air was cool, the street empty. But something in me had changed. I walked to my car slowly, taking in the stillness, the way the moonlight hit the rooftops. I felt both calm and charged – like something had been switched back on inside me.

Wednesday: Ripples

I awoke the next morning with a softness in my chest. The session the night before still echoed inside me. I couldn't stop thinking about the people I'd met, the stories they'd shared, the subtle shifts I'd felt in myself. Everything felt different – heightened, like the world around me had somehow become more vivid. Even the steam rising from my tea felt sacred. I opened my journal and began to write without thinking. Words like 'belonging,' 'truth,' and 'remembering' spilled onto the page. I replayed moments from the circle. The way people nodded when someone spoke their truth. The warmth in the room. Mia's hug.

The card:

You are already on the path. Trust it.

That line wouldn't leave me.

Later that day, I went for a walk. The trees looked greener, the sky more expansive. I found myself at the river – a place I hadn't visited in months. Watching the water glide past, I remembered fishing with my grandad as a child. He used to say, "Silence speaks loudest if you let it."

So, I stood in silence. No headphones. No phone. Just me and the river.

In that stillness, something softened inside me. I realised how rarely I gave myself permission to just be. To feel. To exist without needing to produce, fix or plan. Tears welled – not from sadness, but from recognition.

That evening, I lit a candle and placed the card beside it. I sat cross-legged on the floor and simply breathed. I didn't try to meditate. I didn't follow a script. I just allowed myself to be.

Almost instinctively, I whispered: "Thank you for yesterday. I'm open to whatever comes next."

And for the first time in years, I meant it.

Thursday: A sign

I woke early, the edges of sleep still clinging to my thoughts. As I stretched and opened the curtains, a soft golden hue coloured the sky – the kind that makes everything feel significant. There was a subtle invitation in the air to be still. To notice.

After breakfast, I went for a walk. Something pulled me towards the park. It wasn't far, but I took the long way, letting the morning unfold slowly. As I entered through the iron gates, the rustle of leaves overhead greeted me like a familiar song. Then I saw it – a robin, perched on the edge of a bench, staring directly at me. My grandad had always said robins were signs.

"Messengers," he called them. "If you ever feel lost, look for the robin."

And there it was.

I stood rooted to the spot. The bird didn't fly away. It stayed just long enough for the weight of its presence to land in my chest. A flood of emotion surfaced – memories, longings, unspoken prayers. Not sadness. Not joy. Just a deep sense of being acknowledged. I sat on the bench, took a deep breath, and closed my eyes. I didn't ask for anything. I just listened.

What came wasn't a message – but a feeling.

A thread of connection that ran from that moment, through the park, back to the circle on Tuesday night, and even further still, to something ancient inside me. That afternoon, I dug out an old notebook I hadn't used in years. It was mostly blank, just a few scribbles and half-formed thoughts scattered across its pages. I began to draw what I'd seen on my walk – the robin, a bench, light spilling through trees. It wasn't perfect. But it didn't need to be. It was mine. It was real.

As the day wound down, I noticed I felt different. Quieter inside. But also, fuller. That night, I lit another candle and wrote in my journal: *I don't know where this path is taking me, but it feels like home.*

Then I closed the book and whispered, "Thank you."

Friday: The message

Friday started slowly. No urgency. No list. Just soft light filtering through the windows, the quiet hush of the flat holding me gently. Around midday, my phone buzzed. A message from a friend I hadn't heard from in months:

I heard you've been going to some spiritual thing. I don't know why, but I felt like I needed to reach out. Would you be willing to do a reading for me?

I paused. I had only just begun to trust my own path. But something in me knew this moment was part of it. I messaged back:

Yes. Come over later if you like.

She arrived that evening, wrapped in a coat too big for her. Her eyes looked tired, like she was carrying the weight of too many yesterdays. We didn't say much at first. I made her tea, lit incense and laid out the cards. The air felt different, as if the space itself knew something important was about to happen.

I took a breath, tuned in and began. What came through felt like a river – memories that weren't mine, emotions deeper than words, images landing with quiet certainty. I wasn't analysing. I was connecting. Not just to Spirit, but to her.

She wept. I did too. Not from sadness, but from recognition. From presence. From being seen.

When it was over, she leaned back, her face softer than when she'd arrived.

"I feel lighter," she said quietly. "Like someone finally sees me."

After she left, I sat for a long time in the dim light. That moment had changed something in me. This wasn't just about cards. This was about presence. About meeting someone in their truth. About connection.

Saturday: Reflections

Saturday arrived with a gentle stillness, the kind that invites introspection rather than boredom. I had no plans and, for once, that felt like a gift.

I wandered down to the canal with my sketchbook. The air was brisk, and the water shimmered in the afternoon light. I found a bench and watched the world unfold – cyclists gliding past, a couple walking hand-in-hand, the gentle ripples catching glints of sun. This was the same canal where my grandad used to take me fishing. I hadn't thought about that in years, but as I sat there, I could almost hear his voice – patient, steady, always letting the silence do most of the talking.

I opened my journal and began sketching. Not the robin or the bench this time, but the dream I'd had the night before. A circular room, filled with cushions and candles. People laughing and crying in equal measure. A place where healing didn't need words.

A sanctuary.

The drawing was rough, but it held something. It didn't need polish; it needed truth.

Later, I ran a hot bath and let the water hold me. I thought about the week – how much had changed in such a short time. I felt like a plant that had been growing roots underground without realising and now the first green shoot had broken through.

That night, I journaled again. The word 'connection' came up again and again. Connection to myself. To others. To Spirit. To breath. To memory.

I wasn't learning something new.

I was remembering what I'd always known.

Sunday: Listening

Sunday night, the stars were out in full force. I stood in the garden, wrapped in a blanket, a hot drink warming my hands. I looked up. The sky stretched endlessly above me, stars flickering like sparks of possibility.

"If I'm meant to help people, show me how," I whispered.

My voice was soft. Steady. No thunder. No voice from the clouds. Just the same warmth in my chest that I'd felt with the robin. With the reading. With the river. A quiet knowing.

And then, a memory: My grandad beside me on the riverbank, saying,

"Just listen, son. You'll know what to do."

That was enough.

I stayed outside a while longer. Not seeking answers. Just being. The cold air didn't bother me. I felt held – by the stars, by Spirit, by something far greater than I could name.

Later, I returned inside and wrote in my journal:

I think this is what faith feels like. Not certainty. Just trust.

And underneath that, almost without thinking, I added one word: *Connection.*

Monday: Quiet preparation

There was a stillness in the air on Monday that I didn't want to disturb. I felt like I was in the quiet space between breaths, between what had been and what was still becoming.

I spent the morning cleaning. Not just tidying, but intentionally clearing space. I moved furniture slightly, smudged the corners of each room, opened the windows wide to let the old energy go.

I made soup – slow and nourishing. Chopped vegetables with care, stirred with presence. It felt like a ritual. Even in the simplicity of cooking, I felt it again – that same thread of connection. Between nourishment and care. Between intention and energy.

After lunch, I lit candles and placed the oracle card from that first night back on my altar:

You are already on the path. Trust it.

I smiled. I was starting to.

The afternoon drifted by gently. I played soft music. No phone. No outside noise. Just the flicker of candlelight and the rhythm of my breath. I journaled again.

The words came softly:

Something is unfolding. I don't need to force it. I just need to stay open.

And then, across the page in large letters, I wrote: *Connection.* Because that was the thread I'd been following all along. I went to bed early, knowing tomorrow would bring another step.

Tuesday: The threshold

I returned to the group, changed. What struck me most was how deeply I had felt a sense of connection from the very first evening. Even though this was only my second session, something had already settled inside me. The way we held space. The quiet understanding between strangers. It felt ancient. It was as though I had finally stepped into a place that had been waiting for me all along.

Mia welcomed us back, and I took my seat like someone who had crossed into new terrain. The others seemed different too – softer, more open. As though we'd each gone through something unseen but shared.

That evening's session was gentle. We opened with stillness. Mia guided us into a meditation that felt like returning to the centre of ourselves. No agenda. Just presence. When we emerged, she invited us to share anything that had come up over the week. I listened as others spoke – some quietly, others with emotion. Then it was my turn.

I shared everything. The reading with my friend. The robin in the park. The sketchbook. The stars. The dream of the sanctuary. The door I kept drawing.

And most of all, the connection I now carried – to Spirit, to others and to myself.

Mia smiled, "Sometimes, the week in between is where the real work happens."

The group nodded. And I did too.

As we closed the circle, Mia asked us each to speak one word to capture what we were taking from the evening.

Mine was: Connection. And I meant it. The week had been a return. Not to who I was. But to who I had always been beneath the noise. It was the quietest revolution. One that changed everything. Not by force. But by presence. This wasn't the end. It was a threshold. And I was ready to step through it.

Chris Stanley: www.thesoulalignmentacademy.com

UNBLOCKING YOUR HIDDEN STORIES:

How might this story link to your own experiences?

In which parts of your life would you like to develop stronger connections?

5

UNDERSTANDING

Angie Hayes

We understand abstract concepts best when they are shared as stories. Through storytelling, ideas become relatable, memorable, and easier for the mind to grasp. When we're young, stories help us make sense of the world. In particular, they help us to understand how relationships work. From those early narratives, we begin to shape our sense of self and identity. For many of us, as we grow up, those stories become part of our constantly active inner voice: observing, judging, recording, and interpreting everything around us, all day long.

Michael Singer explores this ever-present chatter in *The Untethered Soul* and Eckhart Tolle affirms the power of peace and presence in *The Power of Now*. That inner voice, rooted in our more primitive brain, is constantly spinning stories, shaped by beliefs, experiences, emotions and perspectives. But we don't have to accept everything that inner voice tells us.

What matters more is deepening our understanding of our true selves: our desires, values and the kind of lives we want to create. When we build this foundation of self-awareness, we become better equipped to quieten that inner voice and respond to the stories it tells with clarity instead of confusion.

This shift is key, especially when dealing with imposter syndrome. Rather than staying stuck in old patterns, we can begin to write new narratives for ourselves, focused on possibilities rather than problems. This is where solution-focused therapy becomes so powerful – it helps us move forward with intention. As in this story, there can be occasions where a more analytical approach may be required to get to the heart of a problem when a client may be struggling to figure something out about themselves. This is where adopting a more integrative approach can produce worthwhile results.

Here, Angie shares an anonymised story of one of her clients, and how, together with Angie, she navigated the stormy waters of imposter syndrome to build a new and more empowering story.

Taming the Imposter

The weekend

Friday evening, 5:30pm and Emily decided it was time to close the laptop and finish for the weekend. She was looking forward to taking a short break for a few days with Sarah and Vicki. The three had been friends for almost forever and, in recent months, Emily had felt much more comfortable opening up to them about what had been going on in her life and how she had been feeling. She felt particularly free with Sarah, who she had known since junior school.

Emily smiled to herself as she made her way to the car, pleased in at least one respect today. She had met her deadline and sent the report to Alison on time. Not only that, she had resisted the urge to procrastinate and obsess about every aspect of it having to be perfect.

She had been in this role for about five months and she absolutely loved it. She was back where she belonged, doing a job she loved and one that she had eventually come to realise that she was actually bloody good at! She congratulated herself for grabbing the opportunity when it presented itself, even if she really hadn't felt like pursuing it at the time. Well, that was one of my better decisions, she mused to herself as she started the car for the journey home.

She thought about what a great boss Alison was. Firm and professional, yet fair, always taking a keen interest in her team.

She was a far cry from the previous bosses Emily had reported to, especially that horrid Brienne. Now, she felt able to discuss her imposter feelings with Alison without judgement. Alison was highly supportive, taking time to check in with Emily on her progress, setting clear expectations and giving Emily the opportunity to be heard and recognised.

As she pulled onto her driveway, Emily continued to express gratitude for everything that had gone so well over the past five months. Having a great job, a great boss, sleeping so much better, becoming more confident and motivated. As she closed the front door behind her, she looked forward to a relaxing evening before the weekend break away with her friends. *I think I deserve a nice glass of prosecco*, she thought to herself, heading for the fridge before fishing a flute glass from the cupboard.

It had been a glorious sunny day, and it was warm still. *Summer is definitely on its way*, she thought as she sat on her balcony looking out towards the sea. She sipped the prosecco and let out a long, luxurious sigh. She had loved this apartment from the moment she walked in and felt truly privileged to live in such a beautiful part of the world and to be blessed with this glorious sea view.

She smiled as she imagined her therapist, Karen, in response to her thoughts, asking "What did it take for you to get here?"

She knew Karen would encourage her to recognise her strengths. How hard she had worked to get here and how much career success she had achieved to enable her to afford this wonderful home.

As she continued to muse, Emily noticed that, irritatingly, other random thoughts had started to pop into her head. *Had she remembered to put that key data into her report? Had she performed a final spell check before she submitted it?*

No! I'm not going down this route again, she told herself firmly. "FFS! Seriously?" She said it quietly, so that her neighbours wouldn't think she'd either lost it or had too much to drink already. *For goodness' sake, Emily! What is WRONG with you?! You've faced so many issues you wouldn't have dreamt of dealing with a year ago. You've completely turned your working life around.*

You're so much happier and noticeably more confident than you have been in ages. Yet here we are, still succumbing to feelings of not being good enough, not being the perfect person in every bloody aspect of life. ENOUGH!

Emily decided distraction was the best remedy for this nonsense. A nice shower, a bite to eat and a bit of packing for the weekend ahead should do it.

These distractions certainly helped. Emily switched her focus to the weekend ahead. The prosecco was chilling in the fridge and she'd done most of her packing. Most of all, she was looking forward to spending quality time with her best friends. It was something she felt she didn't do often enough.

She awoke to the 8:30am alarm, feeling totally relaxed after a great night's sleep, and decided to allow herself a little bit of a lie in after her busy week. When she finally got up, she busied herself with packing the last few things and eating a quick breakfast before the girls arrived to pick her up. She double-checked her packing list to ensure she hadn't missed anything as the doorbell rang. *Oh my God, I'm so anal at times!* she chuckled to herself as she pulled open the front door.

"Oh, my darling, how wonderful to see you!" Sarah exclaimed as she burst through the door, arms outstretched.

Instantly, Emily was wrapped in a wonderful bear hug. Sarah always gave great hugs, and Emily savoured every moment of being held tight, feeling the love and support of her best friend. It gave her an instant lift. Vicki was close behind. She gave Emily a knowing look.

"I had to endure that thirty minutes ago," she said in her usual matter-of-fact way.

Despite their differences, Sarah and Vicki were alike in many ways. Sarah had always been larger than life, finding the positive in everything and never letting anything get her down. She exuded confidence in just about every situation. Always authentically herself, she had a canny way of connecting with people and knowing when it was time to reign in her exuberance.

Vicki was much more reserved. She was self-confident but didn't feel the need to fit in with others who weren't on her wavelength. She didn't make a big deal of it but would quietly and calmly disassociate from anything she felt didn't serve her sense of self-worth. Underneath it all, Emily knew that, despite her protestation, Vicki would have enjoyed Sarah's hug thirty minutes ago just as much Emily was savouring it now.

Emily admired her two friends for their confidence and sense of self-worth. They were, each in their own way, beautiful souls that Emily knew she could trust completely. When the chips were down, they were always there. Their love and support were guaranteed through good times and bad. They were Emily's tribe.

"Right, enough of this nonsense, you two," Vicki said with a huge smile.

She gave Emily a quick no-nonsense hug and a kiss on the cheek. "It's wonderful to see you, hun. Now, we really need to get on the road. There's fun to be had, wine to be drunk and loads to catch up on."

On the way out to Vicki's car, the discussion turned to the weekend.

"What's the first thing you want to do when we get there?" asked Sarah.

Emily replied with her usual, "I really don't mind. You know me, I'm just happy to be spending time with you."

"No," Vicki replied. "You've had a tough year, my girl. This weekend is about taking time out together and giving you a well-deserved chill. So, what would you like to do?"

"Hmm...well... I wouldn't mind a spot of lunch followed by a glass of wine and a chill in the hot tub," Emily responded hesitantly.

"Sounds perfect," Sarah chimed in, as they loaded their bags and headed for their destination.

They weren't going far, only a 45-minute drive out of town and down the coast to a glorious and welcoming spa resort with individual self-contained log cabins, each with its own hot tub and sea view. They arrived in good time, unpacked and looked out across the ocean, breathing in the peace and tranquillity.

Sarah had noticed that Emily had been quiet on the journey down. Nothing too obvious, but Sarah knew her so well. Vicki had picked up on it too. The friends dispatched Emily to the reception area to check out lunch options.

Sarah seized the opportunity. "Is it me Vik, or did you notice that Em doesn't seem quite herself?"

"Yes, I thought the same. We need to get to the bottom of this. She's been through enough turmoil with two job changes and all the stress of the past year. I thought she was loving her new job?"

"I think she is. I wonder if it could be something else. Anyway, let me lead on this. I'll introduce the subject casually. We don't want this to come across as the Spanish Inquisition."

"What are you suggesting?" Vicki asked in mock surprise.

"I think you know exactly what I mean," Sarah smiled knowingly at her friend.

"You know me so well," Vicki laughed.

After lunch, they settled in for an afternoon of relaxing bliss. The hot tub was just the right temperature, warm and welcoming. They relaxed under the warm sun with the sound of the ocean gently ebbing and flowing in the background. Each had a glass of prosecco in hand and all three laughed a lot as they caught up on each other's news. Vicki had been dating a new guy she met online. It didn't take long before the sounds of hilarity cut through the tranquillity of the log cabins, as Vicki recounted the series of disastrous dates that had ensued.

"Are you disappointed, hun?" Sarah asked.

"Not really," Vicki replied. "I take the approach that the first few dates are an introduction to what might lie ahead; not as dates with my soul mate. And this was DEFINITELY an experience to leave behind," she said, as they burst into fits of giggles again.

Sarah had been married to Jason for the past two years. Their wedding had been in the Dominican Republic, partly because they both loved it there and partly because it meant that only those closest to them were in attendance, which was exactly what they wanted. There was a dysfunctional element to Sarah's family, and she had a superb ability to manage their access to her energy and happiness. Jason was keen to start a family, and she now regaled her friends with their conversations about planning when the best time might be and scheduling in time to 'practice.' As usual, Sarah embellished her account to a sufficient degree to make it plausible yet hilariously funny.

"So, come on then, Ems, how are things with you? How's that wonderful new job going?" Sarah asked casually.

Emily's response was unexpected. The hilarity suddenly disappeared as Emily broke down into quiet, dignified sobs. Sarah put her glass down and rushed to the other side of the hot tub to wrap an arm around Emily's shoulder.

"What on earth is the matter, hun? Please don't say it's the new job. We thought everything was going so well." Vicki had moved closer to comfort her friend too.

Emily managed to compose herself. "I'm sorry girls. I'm honestly not sure where that came from, and I don't want to spoil our time together talking about this. The job is great, I'm back in broking, doing what I love. I have a supportive boss and great work colleagues."

"Em, we've known you for years and we know when something is up," Vicki asserted.

"We're all in this life thing together. Fuck the weekend! What's more important is us helping you to get to the bottom of this as much as we can."

"So, the time you spent with your therapist... has that helped?" Sarah asked.

"Of course, it helped enormously! If I hadn't worked with Karen, I would never have made any changes at all. I would still be stuck in that awful, toxic environment with that bloody woman as my boss."

"Oh yes. The infamous Brienne," Vicki smiled.

Emily managed a small smile. "Yes, Karen always used to refer to her as Biryani."

In that moment, the hilarity was restored and the tension in the air began to ease.

"Right then, Em. How did that experience of going to see Karen help you? If you think back to the first time you started working with her to where you are now, what would be the key things you can take away from the experience?"

"That's a great question Vicki," Emily responded. "When I first started seeing Karen, I was a nervous wreck. My anxiety was through the roof, and my confidence and self-worth were at an all-time low."

"So, what was it about that experience that turned things around? What's the most important thing you learned, do you think?"

"I gradually came to realise that I'm prone to people-pleasing. Because of that, I try to fit in with people and situations. Karen helped me to see that the problem wasn't necessarily with me but that the environment wasn't a good one for me. The experience taught me to hold out for my self-worth and to direct my courage towards setting appropriate boundaries at work. I would persistently reach out to colleagues and make an effort to be friendly with absolutely no reciprocity. Karen helped me to understand that it wasn't a personal issue but most likely a cultural issue."

"Well, that seems to have helped. You've moved on in leaps and bounds on that front, hun."

"Yes, I feel I have. I remember when I felt I had to leave the next job after only six months. I was mortified that I couldn't stick it out and I was more worried about what people would think rather than honouring my health and sanity. When I arrived at Karen's, do you know the first thing I said?"

"What?"

"You're probably going to be really annoyed with me, but I've applied for another job."

"What did Karen say?"

"She said, 'Annoyed? Are you mad? I'm bloody ecstatically happy and so proud of you! Good for you.' Then she asked me a great question which has resonated with me since, and I guess it answers your question."

"What was that?" enquired Vicki.

"She asked me, what were the top three things this whole experience had taught me about myself."

"WELL?" Vicki asked with mock impatience.

"It taught me that I'm passionate about what I do, and I don't doubt how capable I am any longer. I've learned to recognise that my own needs are important and to hold out for what I want and need. And, I've now developed a toolkit that helps me to manage my imposter feelings."

"That's fantastic, hun. And we can certainly see the change in you. You've achieved so much success, and you're so highly regarded at work. So, what's going on now, my darling? Why did you burst into tears just now despite having been through so much and getting the outcome you wanted?" Sarah interjected.

"Honestly, I'm not quite sure. All I know is that, at times, my anxiety creeps up, my perfectionist streak rears its ugly head, and I start procrastinating again. All classic signs that my imposter still has a grip on me. I mean, what the hell is wrong with me? As you said, I got the outcome I wanted and still it's not enough."

The tears started stinging Emily's eyes as she spoke her truth.

"Do you think it might be worth going back for another session with Karen? Perhaps she can help you make sense of it? Something is still making you feel unhappy. Perhaps it may not be about work at all?"

"Good point, I hadn't thought of that, Sar. Thank you."

"Right, that's settled," said Vicki as she poured more prosecco into each glass. "Let's drink to our plan. Ems will get in touch with Karen when we get back and we are going to have a great rest of the weekend."

"Cheers!" The three women sang in unison.

Karen's house

Karen finished with her clients for the day and popped her phone off airplane mode to check for messages that needed attending to. She was meticulous about avoiding interruptions when she was with clients.

She had one new message:

'Hi Karen, I hope all is well with you and you are enjoying the sunshine! I just wondered whether it would be possible to book in a session with you over the next few weeks? I have been noticing some familiar traits creeping back in, so I think I'd really benefit from seeing you again. Ideally a Tuesday or a Thursday anytime from 4pm would be great if you can fit me in? Many thanks, Emily xx'

Oh, bless her, thought Karen as she immediately grabbed her diary to look at availability.

'Hi Emily, it's great to hear from you and I hope you're enjoying your new job. Of course, that's no problem. So wise to nip things in the bud. I've got a slot at 4pm next Thursday, if that's any good? Will be lovely to see you x'

It had taken Emily a few days to pluck up the courage to contact Karen. She was torn between wanting to get to the bottom of what was going on and feeling a complete failure.

She arrived the following Thursday at Karen's house. It was great to be back in familiar territory; yet, she felt some trepidation. *I don't know what Karen must think, with me having to come back again*, she thought to herself as she climbed the steps to the front door and looked across at the beautiful view before ringing the doorbell.

Any trepidation immediately vanished.

"Hello, lovely lady. So good to see you!" Karen welcomed her with a warm hug and Emily knew she was back in a safe space.

Sitting in the familiar therapy room, Emily updated Karen on how well the job was going, how well she slotted in, how great Alison was and how she was already doing a full workload and up to speed within five months. When Karen asked what her best hopes were from today's session, Emily opened up about how her imposter feelings were all too present, despite everything going so well on the work front.

"Okay," Karen said confidently. "We're going to get this sorted, don't you worry. As you know, we've been following a solution-focused approach and that's worked well for you so far. But for that final piece of the puzzle, I think we need to get a little more analytical. Are you up for that? Do you trust me?"

"Of course," Emily replied. "What have you got in mind?"

"Let's get to the bottom of this shizzle and look at your core beliefs."

Karen proceeded to ask Emily a series of questions designed to understand exactly how she perceived herself in different situations. Some of the questions were in a category called 'Life in General' and there were two other categories that Emily was free to choose herself. After a bit of thought, Emily chose 'Friendships' and 'Work.' Karen asked a lot of questions and Emily answered each one honestly, knowing that there was no judgement here, just a desire to understand.

Once they had completed the core exercise, Karen played back to Emily some of the thoughts and beliefs she had revealed.

"Do you truly believe that you are this awful?" Karen asked.

"Well, on one level, no, I don't truly believe all of this."

"Good," replied Karen. "Just as I thought. PBB."

"Dare I ask, what on earth is PBB?"

"Primitive Brain Bollocks!"

Emily started to chuckle. You could never stay gloomy for long in these sessions. There was always humour and a good reality check when it was needed. PBB had come up before, so it was timely that Karen reminded her of it now. Emily certainly didn't think that she was as dire as her thoughts led her to believe.

Karen picked out the key themes in Emily's responses and set about asking her why she felt this way about herself and how she might view things differently if that confident version of herself showed up in the room. All the usual suspects were present –

perfectionism, vulnerability, people pleasing, self-worth. Karen picked out another theme, however, that hadn't come up before – comparison to others.

"Exciting stuff," Karen mused. *Not sure I see this as exciting*, Emily thought to herself.

"Let's look at this comparison shizzle. Who are you comparing yourself to and why?"

"I'm not really sure," Emily responded shyly.

"Okay. Would it help to have a little bit of insight while you think about it?"

"Yes please."

Karen proceeded to explain that, in her opinion, it didn't matter what or how we did something if it gave us personal fulfilment and if it didn't adversely impact anyone else.

She then asked Emily, "How will you know when you achieve the success you seek?"

Emily sat in the silence. The silence wasn't uncomfortable. It was Karen's way of giving her time to think and reflect. After a while, something from the last time she'd been here resonated with Emily. She and Karen had discussed how we take on the expectations of others, particularly our parents. Parents are mostly well meaning but, even with the best of intentions, they can instil beliefs. Living out those beliefs and expectations can cause all kinds of problems in adult life until we make the conscious decision to become an adult, set appropriate boundaries and live life on our own terms.

"I think I understand where all of this is coming from," Emily mused, her eyes widening with the realisation of what had been happening. "My Dad always instilled a very strict work ethic into us. You get a good job, then you take the next step up the career ladder, then the next step. You keep striving for a better job."

"Fantastic. So, if I could wave my magic wand and grant you three wishes for this next phase of your life, what three things would be most important to you?" Karen asked.

Emily's response was immediate. "To master my current role and be happy with that for the time being, to spend more quality time with my friends and to have a partner in my life, someone to provide that extra support just for me."

"Wow, and not a greasy pole in sight," Karen responded. "That belief in climbing the career ladder was probably fantastic for your dad. He defined himself by his career success. There's nothing wrong with that, as he clearly found it fulfilling. But is that the life that you want?"

"No, it isn't."

"OK, let's reframe this shizzle within a lovely relaxing trance. Time to get on the couch!"

A restaurant by the sea

It was Saturday evening and Emily was getting ready to go out. She had been looking forward to this moment all day. Ben had suggested dinner at the local Italian restaurant on the seafront. It was one of the better places in town, normally reserved for special occasions.

The doorbell rang and she felt a flutter of excitement. She checked herself in the mirror on her way to the front door. There he stood, ruggedly handsome, with a huge smile on his face and an enormous bouquet of red roses in his hands.

"Evening, gorgeous. You look amazing," he said as he swept in and gave Emily an enormous hug and a lingering kiss on the lips. "Are you ready to go?"

"I certainly am," she responded breathlessly.

When they arrived at the restaurant they were seated at an outdoor table, which meant they could enjoy the view. Emily knew Ben must have planned this date well in advance as tables outside in the summer were like rocking horse poo at this restaurant.

"What time are you and the girls heading off tomorrow?" Ben enquired as he poured two glasses of wine.

"We're not going far so I don't need to leave too early. I expect this will be our last time away for a while before Sarah's baby arrives. I can't believe she's eight months along already."

Ben produced one of his loving smiles. Sarah and Vicki loved him, and he got on so well with both of them, and he and Jason were becoming close friends too.

"How's Vicki doing? How is she getting on with Matt? I may even get to meet him soon at this rate," Ben teased.

"Well," Emily responded, "I'm looking forward to finding out more tomorrow. All I can say is that for Vicki to be dating someone for over six months, that should be a really good sign."

Emily sat back contentedly, looking out to sea, sipping on her wine. *Ben's definitely a keeper,* she thought to herself. *So, this is what it feels like, living life on my own terms. I've become my own person and I'm so excited about what the future might hold.*

Angie Hayes: www.angie-hayes-hypnotherapy.co.uk

UNBLOCKING YOUR HIDDEN STORIES:

Where have you shown others understanding or empathy?

What might help you deepen your understanding of yourself to move forward?

6

HEALING

Debs Penrice

As the last story showed, sometimes people prefer silence over conversation or deliberately tell false stories to mislead themselves or their loved ones. Too many families have hidden stories that remain untold or issues that are never discussed. However, when families keep secrets, the younger generation can suffer from those silences. Perhaps there are hints that the adults are hiding something. Then there are the whispers and gossip that aggravate situations – "She's just like her mother," or "His father was useless, you can't blame him." But no one is brave enough to share the whole story or to talk about it openly. Those silences can create fear and a loss of trust. Or worse, they can affect the listener because they believe the problem is their fault. What we don't always notice is that our children are watching and learning from every move we make. They copy our patterns or rebel against them. The damage this causes is real: without being consciously aware of it, children can repeat the same patterns that their ancestors struggled with – known as ancestral trauma. It also raises the eternal question - which is more powerful, nature, or nurture?

Sharing stories can help us to release those emotions and that generational trauma. Or there are healing methods which explore what's happening in the body without discussing the problems in great depth. Kinesiology is a therapy that uses muscle testing to assess a person's structural, emotional, chemical, or energetic imbalances which may be affecting their physical and mental health. I have had wonderful experiences with two talented kinesiologists and have written this fictional story linked to that healing modality.

A Family Secret

Imogen

The brakes screech and Imogen feels her body fly forward. Bang! The airbag catches her full weight and throws her back into her seat. Next to her, the same has happened to Alex. As she turns her head to check if he's okay, he shouts out, swearing sharply. The car stops and Imogen realises the car behind has rammed into the back of them, but her car has missed the one in front by a whisker's breadth. A small mercy. Imogen gingerly opens the car door and steps out, feeling unsteady as her feet hit the ground. She swaps insurance details with the apologetic driver behind, while Alex calls work to explain his absence; he's going to miss an important meeting. Relieved that the car starts despite the damage to the rear, Imogen has no choice but to drive it home.

Once indoors, Imogen reaches for the kettle, offering to make coffee. But Alex makes his excuses and goes out. Curious as to where he's going, Imogen checks his calendar and notices the only thing marked is lunch at a restaurant in town. Her hands tremor, clutching her mug. She breathes slowly in and out to calm herself as she thinks over the last few weeks. He's been acting strangely for a while.

I know what I can do, maybe Louise is free? She calls her kinesiologist on the off-chance there's an appointment free today. There's no answer, so she types a quick text asking Louise if there's an appointment available at short notice.

When Louise's reply arrives, Imogen is making a cup of tea.

'If you can come over now, I can fit you in – I have a gap in 30 minutes for an hour.'

She grabs a travel mug and heads out. The clinic is walking distance and Imogen can make it over there in twenty-five minutes at a brisk pace. Louise answers the door with a smile and takes her coat.

"Let's get you lying down on the couch and you can tell me what's happening."

"We had a car accident this morning. Nothing serious, but I'm a bit shaken up. Alex rushed off to work anyway, and for me, that set off alarm bells. He's got a mysterious lunch in his calendar. That's all."

As she holds Imogen's wrist gently, Louise is working down each side of her and across her body without touching her. "Mmhmm. But your gut feeling is telling you something is wrong and I'm sensing there's fear trapped in your kidneys and bladder system."

Imogen feels a tear roll down her cheek, as she waits for Louise to say more. "Your adrenal glands feel sensitive too. What else is going on?"

"My mum hasn't been well. Dad is doing his best to cook for her and keep the house tidy, but I've been going over every weekend to help them. It's not too far to drive."

"Have you had any time for yourself?"

"Only to go to the gym. But it's too easy to open a bottle of wine and stop on the sofa for a drink or two in the evenings."

Louise finishes her treatment and talks to Imogen about what might be causing the fear.

"Your kidneys are bearing some additional tension, possibly related to the alcohol. I sense your body is reacting to a deep fear of betrayal or infidelity. Apart from you and Alex, how well are your parents getting on together?"

"Happy enough, I guess. They never really talk about their relationship."

"Is this the first time you've been concerned about you and Alex?"

"Yes, it really is. The more I think about him being secretive, the worse I worry that I missed something important. But I'm sure it's fairly recent."

"Whatever is causing your body to hold onto it, I've released it for today and I recommend a Bach Flower Remedy called Aspen to relieve the fears. I'll give you a few drops now, if that's okay. You need rest and some free space to release this. Maybe a walk?"

"Thank you."

As she leaves Louise's, Imogen calls her mum. "How are you feeling today, Mum?"

"Much better. I caught the bus into town if you're free and have time to meet me?"

Surprised, Imogen answers yes and arranges where to meet. Her work can wait and she's still enjoying the calm after her session with Louise. She catches a bus into the centre and gets off near the coffee shop. Walking in, she spots her mum already seated at a table near the window.

"Hi Mum, how lovely that you're out and about again."

"Yes dear. I was determined to get out from under your father's feet. He's been rather stressed looking after the meals and the shopping. So, I thought I could pick up a few bits and see you at the same time."

"But how could you have known I'd be off work? It's only because we had a bump in the car early this morning; I changed my day around."

"Oh well, it seemed like a good plan to persuade your father I could go out. And we never get time to chat without him listening, so although I'm sorry to hear about the car accident, I'm pleased you're here."

"Great. Mum, I'll order the coffees on the app – what would you like?"

"Oh, just a tea please love – an ordinary cuppa with milk will be fine."

As Imogen concentrates on ordering their drinks, she wonders about telling her mum everything from her appointment with Louise.

"Great, sorted. Mum, I need a bit of help. Alex has been acting a bit strange, and he's not told me who he's going out for lunch with today. Usually if it's a potential client, he can't wait to say there's an opportunity in the making."

"Best not to ask too many questions love. Men don't like a Spanish Inquisition!"

"Surely, it's important to be honest and open in our relationship. You and dad always have been."

"That's not entirely true love. There's never been a good time to tell you before. But it was on my mind last week while I was recovering…"

Imogen stares at her mum, as the waitress puts their drinks down and smiles before leaving them in peace.

"What, Mum? What is it?"

"Well… It turns out, your father was adopted. Your grandmother was not genetically related to you. But I only recently found out because he has been keeping it secret since he learned of it."

"You are kidding me? When did he tell you? Why is this the first I'm hearing of it?"

"Because we wanted it to not affect you. You had a great relationship with your grandmother up until she passed away five years ago. I didn't want to spoil that."

"What do you mean? What else are you not telling me?"

"Your grandmother lied because the adoption was not done entirely through the correct channels. She was worried about getting into trouble or your father being taken away from her. Your father told me about three months ago, but he's known since her funeral."

"So, you've been hiding it for three months? And he's been keeping it secret for five years?"

"I didn't want you to think badly of your grandmother or your father. He's a good man… but his biological mother was an alcoholic and was into low-key thieving to pay for her habit. She died young after having your father."

Imogen slumps back in her seat, the thought of her wine bottle on the counter at home making her shudder.

"I had no idea."

"We don't know much either, but it seems your biological grandmother drank so much because her high-school sweetheart

– your dad's father – cheated on her so frequently. Your father doesn't even know who his biological father was, because she didn't name him on the birth certificate."

Too many questions circle Imogen's mind and she can't figure out which one to ask first. Silence reigns, as Imogen sips her coffee, and her mum stirs the tea to cool it down.

Alex

Arriving late in the office, Alex speaks to his assistant. "I've got an important lunch. Please can you re-arrange everything that was scheduled for this afternoon? I have some gaps on Friday you can use."

Laurel smiles at him, "Of course Alex. No problem. I've sent you the files over too. All edited, ready for you. Are you okay?"

He smiles back brightly, dismissing her question, and walks purposefully to his desk. Work absorbs his full attention as he reads the files and replies to his clients. He sends an apology to the client he missed that morning; no need to give too many details. When the clock strikes noon, Alex gets up, grabbing his coat and laptop bag to head out.

"See you tomorrow, Laurel. Thanks for your help to reschedule everything."

Not waiting to hear her reply, he strides out the door and makes his way to the florist around the corner. He chooses long stemmed orange roses, waiting while the shop girl wraps them.

"These make a beautiful gift, not too romantic," she assures him, while she ties the ribbon.

Alex wonders if he should've picked pink or red. But he pays and scoops them up; he'll be late if he doesn't leave straight away.

Arriving at the restaurant, he hurries away from the doorway to meet the waitress and find his table. He's shown to one directly in the window.

"Ah, please could you move us further back? Great view, but it seems cosier nearer the kitchen. I'm feeling chilly today."

"Certainly sir, is this one more suitable?" she asks, showing him to a seat in the heart of the restaurant.

"Thanks, that's much better," he says, taking his coat off as she offers to hang it up.

Alex fiddles with his tie then checks his phone while he waits. He glances up and sees Zoe walking over to the table, as stunning as he remembers. Wavy, blonde hair, cut a lot shorter than it was when they were students. He stands awkwardly, knocking the chair a little, and offers her the roses.

"Hello. How are you? It's so great that you got in touch," he rambles. She smiles, takes off her coat then accepts the flowers and leans in to kiss his cheek.

"It's been far too long, but I knew you had moved here. So, when my office sent the location for this week's video shoot, I couldn't ignore the co-incidence, could I?" Another smaller smile: he guesses she knows he doesn't believe in co-incidences.

Their conversation flows more easily as they order lunch and eat. Her choice of a chicken burger and chips contrasts with his healthy high-protein salad.

Alex can't help but ask her, "Sounds like you've loved growing in your career. Do you ever wonder 'what if' we hadn't moved to different cities when we first set out?"

Zoe tucks her hair back behind her ears and replies, "No. I don't wonder. I know we would have been good together. But I didn't want to be in London that young. There was just as much opportunity for me in Manchester."

"Yes, well I got tired of London pretty quickly, funnily enough. And here I am in the smallest Oxfordshire market town. Almost settling down."

"You're not married yet?"

"I proposed and she said yes. We're talking through plans to get married next Spring. But..." Alex goes quiet while he scrutinises Zoe's face. Not a flicker.

"Well, it sounds like you met someone lovely."

"Imogen. Yes, she is lovely. But we're not here to talk about her, are we?"

He picks up his glass and takes a slow drink, as he watches her closely again. He feels rewarded when a faint blush reaches her cheeks. Then he remembers the shock of the car accident and Imogen's surprise, as he left the house like nothing had happened. His cheeks burn, as he gazes into Zoe's eyes. Alex focuses back on his lunch, trying to figure out how to break the awkward silence. Zoe smiles playfully and beats him to it.

"Remember that day we got that temp work, helping on an exhibition stand?"

"Yes, we knew nothing about tech, but they had us making non-alcoholic cocktails and we were the busiest stand all day!"

"And it was your idea to carry on to the bar for real cocktails afterwards. I think we spent most of the cash we earned, didn't we?"

He laughs. He still loves an occasional mojito even now. As if she read his mind, Zoe leans in across the table.

"So, are we going out tonight, or what? I'll be finished by 8pm."

Alex feels his stomach churning. He nods but can't find any words. Sitting opposite Zoe again, the years fall away, and the rush of energy makes him straighten in his seat.

Imogen

Opening the door to the empty house, Imogen makes more tea and then sits at her desk, intending to do some work. She has a deadline. But she can't stop thinking about her dad's adoption and Alex's mysterious lunch.

She forces herself to concentrate. This presentation won't create itself and she's got a wonderful new client who she wants to share team well-being ideas with, at their workshop next week. They're a video production company, growing fast. They hired her because they've never had a HR director, yet they're keen to take care of their people and build a great culture. She heard they have a shoot in her area this week, but so far, the on-location film team haven't been in touch. She writes, adds images, and analyses data from the employee survey they'd done together. Her phone distracts her, and she smiles because it's Alex. Her smile quickly fades again:

'Too much work to catch up on – will be late. Don't wait for me to eat. A x'

She turns back to her work. But feeling a pang of hunger, Imogen realises she's worked straight through, and now it is late afternoon, with the sky darkening.

She steps outside and breathes in the Autumn smell of damp leaves. She thinks of Louise, reminding her to make space to rest. It does feel restful out here and she stays there until the sun is setting. How many times had she and Alex watched the sun set together?

Alex

Zoe had left for her late afternoon video shoot. He wanders along the high street, unsure where to go to kill the time in between. He has plenty of work to get through, if he can find a quiet space. Yet the coffee shops are all heaving and closing soon.

Why not go home? But if he does, it'll be almost impossible to go out again and meet Zoe for drinks later tonight.

Does he even want to? He texts Imogen before he can change his mind.

He walks past the library and notices they're open late. Perfect: it's quiet and he's unlikely to bump into anyone he knows. The desks upstairs are empty. He chooses one and settles in to prepare for Friday's meetings. Finishing one set of files, he notices the horizon darkening outside. He feels peaceful as he thinks of the sunsets he's watched over the last three years, by the sea, on hillsides and in the forest – with Imogen. Shoving his laptop into the bag, he jumps up and heads out of the library.

Home

Imogen walks back into the kitchen after her makeshift dinner, reaching for a glass in the cupboard. It's not quite 8pm and she hesitates by the wine glasses, before picking a tumbler instead. She mixes cordial with tap water, then pours the rest of the red wine down the sink.

The front door bangs. She hears Alex in the hallway, then he's beside her in the kitchen. He notices what she's done and takes the bottle gently out of her hand. He wraps his arms around her and hugs her tight.

Debs Penrice: www.storyhealing.net

UNBLOCKING YOUR HIDDEN STORIES:

Which shared moments have led to stories being created in your family?

How might they unlock inspiration for others?

7

RESPECTING

Caroline Smith-Mclean

When a character in a story does something we admire, we respect them. When a friend stands their ground for what they believe in, we respect them too. What we respect in others helps us to figure out our own values and who we want to be. Yet, few of us offer ourselves the self-love and respect that we extend to others.

The relationships we have with other people are often like mirrors. They reflect back to us the parts of ourselves that are still raw, unhealed or hidden. We can be triggered, hurt or deeply moved by that which requires our attention. Yet, we rarely understand what it's showing us. Instead, we tell ourselves stories; stories that tell us that we are responsible for the behaviour of someone else, or worse – that we are to blame.

Understanding and respecting our own true nature is a key step on the journey to healing. In this story, Caroline Smith-Mclean shows how relationships in which we want and hope to feel safe can sometimes transform into relationships that threaten our sanity and self-worth. She says, "We make ourselves wrong. We believe we're responsible for their behaviour. We absorb blame that was never ours to carry. And those internal stories, those little voices in our heads, can be the most damaging of all. But here's what I know for sure: healing begins when we shift the narrative. Respecting our boundaries, our worth, is where real transformation starts. The relationships that challenge us the most are often the ones holding up the biggest mirror, showing us exactly where we have given our power away."

Thankfully, we have tools and healing modalities to help us overcome these negative patterns, escape these kinds of relationships and build new connections founded on self-respect, self-belief and self-love. Stories of overcoming can powerfully reflect our need for self-love and self-respect.

Finding the One

She was sixteen, sitting on the edge of her bed, anticipation buzzing through her veins.

Any minute now, he would arrive to pick her up. She had straightened her hair until it was sleek and smooth, applied just enough makeup to make her eyes stand out, and finished with a delicate spray of J'adore on her wrists and neck. The scent felt like a promise, a whisper of romance, of being wanted.

Her phone buzzed. Her heart leaped. She grabbed it, a small smile on her lips.

"Hi Babe," she said.

"Hey, sorry, I'm not picking you up today. I'm on my way to pick up my girlfriend."

She laughed at first. A knee-jerk reaction. *What kind of messed-up joke was this?*

The air in the room suddenly seemed too thin.

Her fingers gripped the phone tighter, her pulse drumming in her ears.

"Wait...what?"

But the line was already dead.

For a moment, she sat there, staring at the screen. Confused. Trying to process the words he had spoken so casually. Her guy, the one who had whispered about their future, about meeting his mum, about getting married one day, had just erased her.

Like she was nothing.

Then the punch to the stomach. A violent wave of nausea surged through her. She barely made it to the bathroom before she was on her knees, heaving; her entire body trembling as the reality set in. It wasn't a joke.

The stories flooded in, crashing over her like the incoming tide.

What did I do wrong? Why wasn't I enough? Why did he change his mind all of a sudden? How can I convince him it's me he wants?

Not once did it occur to her, this isn't your fault. Not once did she think, you deserve more than this.

By the time she got to college the next day, she was hollow. The pain clung to her like a second skin. She couldn't eat, couldn't focus.

That night and the next and the next, her mind raced, playing their last conversations like scenes from a movie, searching for the moment she had failed. Searching for proof that she was defective, unworthy, disposable.

Heavy, painful tears were now her constant companions. And then came the thought.

A way out.

She picked up the tablets. One by one, she took the entire blister pack, barely tasting them, barely thinking beyond the crushing weight in her chest.

Maybe this was the only way through the pain. Or maybe...just maybe...someone would finally see how much she was hurting and fix it for her.

But...she felt the guilt of doing this to her family. She heard her dad, walking down the hallway, whistling. She called to him. His face turned pale; his voice thick with panic.

The next thing she knew, they were at the hospital, where the nurses moved quickly.

A cup of charcoal was pressed into her hands. She drank it down, the bitterness coating her throat, but nothing could dull the pain inside.

No charcoal could fix what was broken. They asked her "Why" and told her that no man was worth this.

They spoke about the possibilities of long-term effects. Not just the tablets but that this could be on her record forever.

"Mental health problems," they called it. But nothing happened... nothing changed. She still felt empty.

That was the first crack in the foundation. The first lesson in how little she thought of herself. The first desperate attempt to be seen, to be valued, to be enough. The start of a long journey that would take her through self-sabotage, broken relationships, years of seeking love in all the wrong places. Eventually, to something else.

Something better.

But not yet. First, she had to fall.

Two years passed. Life felt like the best it had ever been. A blur of drunken nights, dimly lit bars, and the bass thumping in her chest and beneath her feet. A new kind of rhythm had taken over her life. Drink, sleep, work, repeat.

On the surface, she knew she looked alluring and sexy. That's what men wanted, right? The red lipstick, the too-loud laugh, the way she threw her head back with reckless abandon. Men watched her, drawn in.

Even when she wasn't drinking, they'd assume she was drunk. So full of life, so uninhibited. This had to be the glow-up, right? Proof that she had risen above the past? Reinvented herself? Except it wasn't.

Beneath the electric buzz of the nightclub lights, beneath the glances exchanged with strangers, beneath the makeup and the laughter, beneath it all, the numbness and emptiness remained. A quiet, aching void that no amount of attention could fill.

She believed one thing, though. If they wanted her body, at least they wanted something. That was better than nothing, right? Right?

Each time a man leaned in close, each time hands traced her skin, a silent hope flickered: Maybe this is it. Maybe this is the one who will make me feel whole.

But morning always came. And with it, the same emptiness. She told herself she was having fun, that she was in control, that she could stop whenever she wanted. But deep down, she knew the truth – she wasn't chasing pleasure.

She was chasing proof. Proof that she was enough. Proof that she was wanted.

Because if someone wanted her, even for just a night, then maybe, just maybe, she wasn't so easy to leave behind.

More years passed. She was getting married. It was her dream. She was chosen. She belonged to someone.

Sure, some things had happened. The break ups. The make ups. The other woman. The distant and avoidant behaviour. The mood swings. The passive aggression.

But now they were exchanging vows to dedicate their lives to each other.

I am the one that someone wants to be with, she told herself as she stepped into her dress. It shimmered in the soft light of her bedroom, the delicate lace catching the sunlight with every movement.

She stood before the mirror, her fingers tracing the intricate pattern, a smile barely grazing her lips, her heart fluttering. She had dreamed of this moment for years. The moment when she finally arrived. She was chosen. Her reflection in the mirror didn't lie.

Outside, the house buzzed with energy. The laughter of bridesmaids, the chatter of children playing, the scent of fresh flowers filled the air.

The wedding was everything she dreamed it would be. The ceremony was perfection itself. The vows, her father's hand steady in her own as he walked her down the aisle. Everywhere was love and joy. They danced the night away, the world fading behind them as they were swept up in the promise of forever.

Finally, she was enough.

Time passed, and the reality of life together settled in. The children, the shared responsibilities, the quiet moments in between. She watched him, her husband, consumed by work. Always "too busy" to do what she wanted to do as a couple or as a family.

Life had changed, but the distance remained. Getting married had not fixed things.

Yes, he was physically present. But he remained emotionally distant, his moods swinging from one extreme to the other, sometimes shutting down completely. He was stressed, he said. Life was hard for him, he explained.

But in the quiet spaces between his words, she wondered, *Where do I fit in?*

He went out with his friends, often without notice, returning at odd hours.

She'd wait for him to come back, to be present with her, to be the man he had promised to be. And yet, she couldn't shake the feeling that something... someone... was slipping further away. The part of her that had dreamed of love, of connection, felt small now.

She was losing herself in the silence, hiding behind her role as wife and mother, telling herself everything was fine. After all, it had to be. *Didn't it?* She was chosen now. *Wasn't she?*

"I need a night out," he said.

He told her he'd had a tough week... pressure from work, stress piling up. She didn't argue. She never argued anymore. She understood. Or at least, she told herself she did.

Midnight came and went... then 3am... and 6am. A familiar knot twisted and grew in her stomach. She lay in bed, still and silent, pulling the duvet tightly around her like armour. But the anxiety crept in anyway, uninvited and persistent.

Where is he?

By 8am, her thoughts were racing too fast to ignore. Her hands trembled as she picked up the phone and called his friends.

"Yeah, I'm sure he's fine," one said casually.

"You know how he is. Probably crashed at someone's house," said another.

Their words didn't settle her. It wasn't fine. It never really was.

At 10am he walked through the door. No apology. No explanation. No eye contact. Just a heavy silence, and a tired face that wouldn't meet hers.

She stood in the hallway. Watched him shuffle past as if she were invisible.

Her throat tightened. Her heart pounded. She felt ridiculous standing there like a statue, but she couldn't move, couldn't make sense of the cocktail of anger, sadness, confusion, and something deeper. Something like grief.

Finally, she found her voice. Fragile but steady.

"I thought you said you'd be home around three?"

He rolled his eyes. "Why are you crying?"

The question hit like a slap. Not asked out of genuine concern. Asked like an accusation. Tears spilled over before she could catch them. She wanted to say she was scared. That she'd spent hours wondering if something terrible had happened. That her mind had spiralled into the darkest possibilities while their children slept. But the words caught in her throat. Instead, she stood there, shaking. "I was just worried," she whispered.

And then came the shame. The guilt. The self-doubt.

Am I overreacting? Should I just let it go? He's home now. He's safe. That's what matters, right?

She stuffed her feelings down like so many times before. She went on with the day. Made breakfast, got the kids ready, went to the park. Smiled when she needed to. But inside, she was somewhere else entirely. Lost in a storm of questions she'd been taught not to ask.

Is it okay to feel like this?

Am I allowed to want more?

Is love supposed to feel this... lonely?

She was there, but not really there. Her body was present. Her heart was elsewhere. She watched her children laugh and wished she could feel that kind of lightness again.

When he finally stirred from sleep and while the kids were distracted, she knew she couldn't hold it in any longer.

"Where were you last night?" she asked softly. Her voice betrayed her, quivering with the weight of everything unspoken.

His expression shifted in an instant. Cold. Defensive. Dismissive.

"Why are you crying?" he asked again. "It's embarrassing that you called my friends," he said, like her concern was some shameful inconvenience.

The words hit her harder than a punch. She flinched but stayed standing.

"I was worried," she whispered, barely audible over the thudding in her chest.

Worried because you didn't come home.

Because you'd promised. Because I don't know where I stand anymore.

The silence that followed wasn't peaceful. It was thick, charged and cruel.

"You said you'd be back at 3am," she added, trying to stay composed even as her throat tightened.

He rolled his eyes. "What's wrong with you? I didn't do anything."

And just like that... it was her fault again. She swallowed the lump forming in her throat, her entire body tensing against the rising tide of emotion.

He was here now, wasn't he? That should be enough. She told herself that. Over and over. But deep down, she knew, it wasn't enough. Not anymore.

She questioned herself.

Maybe I shouldn't have said anything.

Maybe I should've let it go. Am I too much?

He stormed out of the room, frustrated, muttering under his breath. She stood frozen, shaking, tears pouring down her cheeks in a mix of rage, hurt, humiliation. Ten minutes later, he returned and found her still crying.

"What is wrong with you?" he snapped again. "I haven't even done anything. Why are you crying?"

That statement again. I haven't even done anything. It came after every shutdown, every dismissal, every denial of her reality. She wanted to scream, to tell him that his nothing felt like everything. But the words never came.

Instead, she wiped her tears away, swallowed her pain, and got on with the day. She felt like a little girl who'd been scolded for speaking up. Like she'd been shut down for needing something she wasn't supposed to ask for.

A few weeks later, it happened again. The same cycle playing out. Again. And again. Him going out, leaving her feeling all alone, coping with everything alone. In the quiet moments, when the noise of the world faded, her thoughts spiralled, as she replayed a scene, his words, his tone, his complete inability to see her. How often had she stood there, heart wide open, and he slammed the door on it, as if it meant nothing?

That's when the truth started whispering to her. This wasn't just about him. It was about her. It was about the years she had spent shrinking, silencing herself, smoothing over every sharp edge so that she wouldn't be "too emotional." So that she wouldn't be left. So that she could keep the peace. But in doing that, she had abandoned herself.

The worst part was that she hadn't even noticed when it started. It just… happened. Little by little. Until she didn't recognise herself anymore.

This isn't who I am supposed to be.

A question rose up, no longer easy to silence: *Could I change things? Could I finally choose myself without guilt? Without fear dragging me back into the same old dance?*

For years, she had lived with fear. Fear of rocking the boat. Fear of being alone. Fear of not being enough. But the peace she was trying to protect had never really existed. Not truly. It was always a fragile silence, held together by her sacrifices.

But this time felt different. This time, something had shifted. She had been to the edge of the abyss. She had felt the darkness close in and wondered if the light would ever come back.

But then, something shifted. On a friend's advice, she tried coaching and hypnotherapy. Deep work within herself that slowly, quietly, began to tear down the walls she had built around her heart. She wasn't the same woman. It seemed a veil had lifted. For the first time in what felt like an eternity, she saw things as they were, not as she wished them to be.

The fog had cleared, and in its place, a profound clarity blossomed. She was enough. She was worthy of peace, of love that didn't drain her, of a future where she wasn't always second-guessing herself.

She reflected on the years she had spent twisting herself into knots, hoping for a change that never came. Now, she felt something different. A strength rising from the depths of her being. A new sense of power. Slow at first, like a flickering flame. But it was real. Even though she stayed, the more she focused on herself the less she worried about him and his reactions. She felt stronger than she ever had before yet knew she had a way to go.

Yet, as much as she had changed, the world around her remained the same. He remained the same, he wielded his emotional manipulation like a weapon, his every word dripping with the weight of their shared history. Each conversation was a battleground, a war of words designed to bring her back into submission.

"We're not going to just give up after all these years, are we?" he asked, his voice edged with faux sincerity.

"Think of the kids. Think of what you are doing to the kids. You don't want to be that person. You don't want to let them down."

The guilt. The shame. All rushing back, drowning her in waves of self-doubt.

How many times had she been on this precipice, where everything could change, but where the fear crept in, convincing her to stay, to settle, to believe in the illusion he was selling? But this time, despite the rising tide of his words, she didn't flinch.

She could feel the shift within her, a soft but undeniable knowing that no matter what he said, she deserved more than this. Something inside her was waking up. And once she had woken up, it was impossible to go back to sleep.

She wasn't here to live a half-life. She'd discovered a world beyond this and she had a plan. Still, he persisted, his words an arsenal of emotional manipulation.

Tears. Pleas. Desperate proclamations of how much he loved her, how he couldn't lose her, how their family would fall apart if they weren't together. She watched him standing there. And, for the first time, she really saw him.

She didn't just hear the words. Now, she saw the patterns, created over years. The emotional blackmail, the subtle and not-so-subtle threats. She realised how deeply she had been buried under the weight of it all, how much of her life had been dictated by someone else's needs, someone else's fears.

But now she could see. With that vision, something inside her hardened.

Her sense of self, her inner compass, had been rewired. She was no longer a shadow of her former self, clinging to the hope that things would magically get better. She now knew that she was her own person, deserving of a life that was true to her.

A year later, she met a man who treated her right. Who saw her. Chose her. Loved her deeply. Who held her through her silence, celebrated her fire, and showed her what real love felt like. But despite his gentleness and unwavering presence, she still didn't feel safe.

No amount of time together ever felt like enough. She endlessly craved his affection, his words, his gestures. But she couldn't trust them.

She was always waiting for things to change. For the other shoe to drop. For love to leave, just like it had before. She couldn't shake the feeling that it was too good to be true.

So, she pulled away before she could be abandoned. Sabotaged the very thing she'd always said she wanted. Because, deep down, a part of her still believed she wasn't enough to keep it.

None of it was wasted, though. Not the heartbreak. Not the break-up. Not the ache of walking away from something beautiful.

Because that was the moment, the real turning point.

The point at which she stopped waiting for someone else to love her enough to fill the void inside. The point at which she made the radical decision to turn inward. To do the work. To face the patterns. To take accountability. Not blame, but accountability.

To realise that how she'd been treated in the past didn't matter if she didn't also expect more, ask for more, know she deserved more. She knew it sounded cliché. Cheesy even. The kind of thing that used to make her roll her eyes and say, "Ugh, gross."

But this time? It hit different.

Because it was her truth.

She stopped romanticising potential. She stopped settling for scraps of love and calling it a feast. She built boundaries like a queen...firm, unapologetic, sacred.

And now, aged nearly 40...

She'd found the one. The love of her life.

Someone who treated her in a way no one ever had, not because someone else completed her, but because she finally knew her worth.

Her boundaries were strong. Her peace was non-negotiable. Her standards weren't for sale.

And the best part? The person she found...was herself.

She came home. To the woman she was always meant to be. To the version of herself that had always been there. Waiting behind the fear, behind the people-pleasing, behind the pretending.

And damn...what a beautiful homecoming it was.

Because healing isn't just about finding love.

It's about becoming it.

Caroline Smith-Mclean:
www.carolinesmithmcleanhypnotherapy.com

UNBLOCKING YOUR HIDDEN STORIES:

How do you relate to this story of feeling secure?

Where in your life could you develop greater respect for your core values?

8

REVEALING

Gerwyn Tumelty

In contrast, when stories are shared openly, they enable us to reveal or explore parts of ourselves that otherwise might remain hidden in the shadows. But, as explored in the last chapter, we might stay silent or only share that which we feel others will deem acceptable. Or we heavily adapt our stories until they're entertaining or exaggerated for dramatic effect. We might struggle to reveal the true story.

Yet sharing stories with each other after time has passed is one way to defuse the emotions held within. Some people use distractions, different conversations and activities to keep them busy while they process their own stuff. Others spend time alone to process their emotions but continue to work and function in their daily lives. Then there are those who shut themselves completely away because the shadows are too hard to accept, perhaps because they cause fear, anger or shame. A further way to process emotion is through writing. That's how Gerwyn Tumelty decided to approach his experience of trigeminal neuralgia, an extremely painful nerve disorder. The challenge of sharing our truth even with trusted friends is also very real. Yet we all benefit hugely from being listened to and, when given room, from sharing our stories with others. Gerwyn's story explores those moments of space and true connection, when we reveal what had been hidden.

Below the Surface

"It's great that you opened up, Tom. We're always here for you, you know that. But you really need professional help."

Tom and Owen sat starboard on the cockpit of *White Lady*, sharing a bottle of tepid water. Harri had already left for the long drive back to Wiltshire. The 26-foot yacht was secured to a pontoon, as the usual weekend pedestrian traffic moved along the stone walls along the edges of Penarth Marina. Some stared down at the yachts lined up on the pontoons, maybe trying to find answers to life's questions or dreaming of different lives altogether.

Earlier, Tom, Harri and Owen had spent a couple of hours tidying, cleaning and squaring the yacht away. Washing up, wiping down, emptying the bins and taking the waste to the recycling point; stowing the equipment and 'cheesing down' the ropes, as they had all learned to do during their time at sea, now many years ago. Owen's attempt at the ropes had made Harri and Tom smile, as did the usual military banter that the three fell into.

They stowed the small inflatable tender that they had used to replace the emergency life raft pod. It hadn't been the easiest job. Harri, being the tallest, was sent astern to stand in the floating tender, supporting the old pod while Owen and Tom, standing on deck, unbolted it from the guard rails. It would have been funny, but embarrassing too, if Harri had taken a dive into the marina water – as engineer officers in the military, safety had been paramount. They fitted the new pod swiftly and without incident. It was all a welcome distraction for Tom – a little normality after what had turned out to be an emotional weekend.

They had known each other nearly twenty-five years. Harri and Owen were already friends when Tom met them, having completed undergraduate military engineering degrees in Plymouth. Tom got his engineering degree at Bath and joined the military soon after. The three men were driven, ambitious and highly capable and, as they quickly learned in training together, had a lot in common. All three were pragmatic, emotionally intelligent and had a similar sense of humour.

It was no surprise that their wives also got on well. Owen and Harri had met Claire and Vicky while they were all undergrads. Tom had met Sarah in Cardiff where she was studying to be a teacher and he took a master's degree in advanced engineering mechanics. The three girlfriends had enjoyed many social events and get-togethers while their boyfriends were training to become officers. The friendship between the three men, their wives and, in time, their children, continued after the three left the military.

—

Owen's words pushed every other thought out of Tom's head, holding centre stage like the headline act at a music festival. But this wasn't a track Tom had heard before. It was not how he had imagined the weekend would end. He wasn't sure what to think after the two days he'd experienced. They had all been looking forward to the weekend. Now, they would remember it for a very different reason. Tom couldn't help feeling that he was to blame. Heaviness had replaced humour. Laughter had turned to tears and the fun had turned to functionality.

But, sitting there, next to Owen, feeling the kindness of his friend's words, he no longer felt like a liability or a broken part. He no longer felt the loneliness that had engulfed him for the past five years; possibly longer. He had told them. He had shared his story of mental torture and pain. He didn't know what would happen next. But he now knew he had the support and reassurance of his two trusted friends.

—

White Lady was Owen's boat. It was old and he'd been doing it up. When the yacht and skipper were ready for their first shakedown sail – to identify problems, fix what was broken and confirm that his hard work had resulted in a yacht ready for longer trips – Owen asked his two old friends if they'd like to come along as crew for the weekend. It had been a while since they had spent time just with each other, without their families. Owen suggested a meal at the marina restaurant on Friday evening, the shakedown sail on Saturday morning, followed by a walk into Penarth town for dinner on Saturday evening, and back on their respective roads home by lunchtime Sunday.

Owen was already onboard when Tom arrived on Friday evening. He passed Tom a can of chilled lager and gave him a man hug. Tom was grateful for both. It was almost a year since the three families had been to the Dordogne, but it felt as if it had only been a week. Harri arrived soon after to the same welcome.

Over the cans of beer, the three friends caught up. They were all equally proud of their sporty children. Tom shared the news of his oldest son's success representing Wales in the 1500m; Owen glowed as he described his daughters' footballing achievements; and Harri talked about driving his daughter and her horse around the country for equestrian events.

After some more conversation and a few drinks on board, the three quickly changed for dinner and walked up the pontoon to the marina restaurant.

Tom had been quite the beer drinker when he was younger, in the company of his friends and teammates at the rugby club. He no longer drank much but, this evening, the drink was going down easier than normal, and he was starting to feel the effects of the bottles of red wine they had ordered for the table. Foresight as well as hindsight is a wonderful thing, but he was in the moment and enjoying himself.

They talked for hours, about the challenges of being parents and husbands. Tom wondered if their three wives had had a similar conversation during their recent spa weekend. *We can all be difficult to live with*, he thought. By now, Owen and Harri were running through the names of people they had trained or served with. It was a ritual of sorts, sharing news of or wondering what their former friends and colleagues were up to now.

The conversation wound around to their own careers. Maybe it was the alcohol, or something else, but Tom was having difficulty engaging in the conversation and felt somewhat detached, like he was having an out-of-body experience, with his thoughts wandering far and wide. After successful military careers, Owen was now chief engineer at a facilities management company and Harri was chief operations officer for a technology start up. Both clearly enjoyed their jobs, although the pressures were obvious. Tom was proud of what his friends had achieved. He wasn't envious of them, but he sometimes felt inferior.

He had been the first to leave the military, in his late twenties. Having given eight years to Queen and country, he'd been hit by a gut feeling to seek a life outside the services. But his post-military career wasn't without its ups and downs. An unsuccessful attempt to start his own business had led to a stint as a project manager in the energy sector. While the work was lucrative, it was also unreliable, and with three teenage children, a little under a year ago he'd taken a managerial job at a local tech company. The job, however, hadn't lived up to its promise and he knew, almost immediately, that he had made the wrong decision. He was struggling and, as much as he tried to convince himself otherwise, he was deeply unhappy.

It had taken ten years for him to feel that he could confidently contribute to Harri's and Owen's career conversation. When they had trained together, the three friends had been professional equals, but now, in Tom's mind, the others had risen above him.

Staring at the glass of wine cradled in his hand while his friends shared boardroom stories and political power plays, he felt a failure.

At work now, he simply went through the motions – team meetings, programme reviews, technical discussions – thinking that his output was acceptable. One day, about six months into the job, he was invited to a meeting with Steve and Pete, the company owners. Tom looked forward to this meeting as an opportunity to develop his relationship with them, and to demonstrate his ability to operate at director level. He offered a detailed project update, but they told him that was unnecessary. The agenda for the meeting, rather, was Tom's performance. Their feedback confirmed everything he had not wanted to hear.

The meeting affected him deeply – not only what was said, but how they had planned and conducted it. Any remaining hope of building a rapport had sailed away over the horizon, and he was alone. He sat quietly, trying to listen carefully, but his mind raced. He felt paralysed and in shock. He had no defence to offer. Nothing. What made matters worse was they did not ask him for a response. They sought no discussion; nor did they want to understand or help.

The meeting was a warning, and his predicament, coupled with the tone of the meeting, cut straight through him. Since then, he had been replaying and ruminating on that day. It messed with his head and his values, and it exposed something that had long been buried in the depths of his mind.

To his horror and shame, he started to think how much easier it would be to no longer be on this planet, to disappear for good. The suicidal thoughts that he'd not experienced since he'd finally had his surgery nearly three years ago had now come back. He was drowning, struggling to stay afloat. Dropping like a wreck and sinking to the bottom of the ocean, he had no idea how to return to the surface.

The weekend with Harri and Owen seemed like an opportunity to escape, to find an air bubble, to forget his world, his life, his worries. But now he found himself trying his utmost to listen to his friends as they talked about work. He felt as if he was listening to them underwater. He was looking their way, watching them, but he could not hear what they were saying.

The job and the meeting weren't the only things making him feel like a wreck on the ocean floor. But no-one, not even Sarah, knew about the dark places in his mind. If he started to talk about things, who knows where he would stop?

—

Back in the saloon of *White Lady*, with music playing in the background, the conversation and alcohol continued to flow. It was dark now and the lights in the cabin were low. The three friends tried not to disturb the residents of neighbouring yachts but, three sheets to the wind, they were finding it difficult to stay quiet.

Harri was acting DJ, filling the yacht with Brit pop and electro funk. Tom requested *High and dry* by Radiohead, a song that pierced his soul like a knife whenever he heard it. It seemed appropriate for his mood now. Harri raised an eyebrow at this rather sombre choice but played it anyway.

The words resonated in Tom's head: "… you broke another mirror, you're turning into something you are not…."

Picking up on the music, or perhaps on Tom's energy, Harri asked, "How's your head now since the operation?"

The question crashed into Tom like a breaking wave. He couldn't speak. Fine, he wanted to say, but instead stared blankly at Harri. He could no longer hear the music. Was Harri asking about the physical scar or about how he really was? Tom's mind was spinning with flashbacks of physical pain, deep depression, loneliness, mixed with all he'd had to drink since the start of the evening.

Suddenly, the dam of emotions that had been holding since his surgery burst. Tears rolled down his cheeks. There was no stopping the water that came rushing over the sea wall.

—

Four years earlier, Tom had been diagnosed with trigeminal neuralgia, an extremely painful condition that had started out as frequent headaches and then extended into facial pain. He'd found it difficult to describe the tension-like pain to his doctor and dentist. Sometimes dull, sometimes sharp, the pain was triggered by cold drinks and sometimes hot drinks. Sometimes it came on when he was tired, sometimes in the mornings after a good night's sleep. It was unpredictable, but it was always around the jaw joint on the right side of his face. Sometimes he felt it inside the jaw itself, like a deep toothache.

Neither his doctor nor dentist could establish the cause. The pain progressively worsened and, before long, he felt pain every time he ate or drank, like a combination of electric shocks, sometimes in pulses, sometimes continuously, deep in the jaw, under the teeth, episodes lasting from seconds to minutes at a time. Normal painkillers were ineffective. To Tom, it felt like a screwdriver was being pushed into his bone and slowly twisted.

The pain affected his sleep, his moods, his relationships and his ability to work. His nights were interrupted, and the combination of pain and tiredness caused him to grow impatient and short tempered. Sarah and the boys were upset to see Tom suddenly convulse in pain during meals. Tom hated the feeling of helplessness and guilt his pain bestowed on all of them. At work, colleagues and clients had started to notice, wondering why he suddenly walked out of meetings or went home early. As an independent contractor, the pain was having an impact on his earnings.

As his quality of life deteriorated, he started to suffer mentally and emotionally. He began to wonder if the cause was psychological, due to stress or anxiety. He discussed it with his doctor, but the doctor did not know. It was time to explore other options.

After some research and a recommendation from Sarah, Tom met with a therapist.

"Have you considered that it might be trigeminal neuralgia?" she asked Tom.

"Tri what?" he replied. His own online research had not uncovered this very rare condition. He listened intently as the therapist told him about a friend who had symptoms that sounded remarkably like Tom's.

"You'll have to write it down for me," Tom said. As he took the piece of paper with the name on it, he felt a strong sense of hope, like a fog lifting at sea.

Within forty-eight hours, he had searched online and seen his doctor. The doctor had sufficient information to prescribe carbamazepine. The speed at which this drug worked surprised everyone. Trigeminal neuralgia, however, is notoriously difficult to diagnose, as the facial pain could be caused by a myriad of other health problems. It would take almost a year for a consultant to give a definitive diagnosis, but the immediate effectiveness of the carbamazepine would form part of that diagnosis.

The twelve months between discovering he might have trigeminal neuralgia and receiving a formal diagnosis were far from smooth sailing. In fact, Tom was regularly battered by waves of pain. He thought of his trigeminal neuralgia, and his treatment of it, like a mountain range. The mountains were his pain, and the carbamazepine was the flood water filling the valleys.

At first, the mountains weren't particularly big and the peaks were easily flooded by the rising water. But, as the months passed, the mountains grew higher and more water was needed to submerge the peaks, with the doctor increasing the dosage beyond the maximum advised.

That the pain was getting worse was most visible to those closest to him. Sarah tried to keep things as normal as possible for the children as Tom became ever more distant. What his distance masked were his increasingly frequent suicidal thoughts.

Tom spent countless hours online learning about his indiscriminate attacker, working out how it could be effectively disarmed and brought to justice.

A series of tests eventually led to a consultation with a maxillofacial specialist who finally formalised the diagnosis of trigeminal neuralgia. As the consultant confirmed what Tom had known for a year, Tom's eyes filled with tears and he felt the emotional tide rise within him.

He knew the road ahead was still a long one. He was to have microvascular decompression (MVD) surgery, which would involve more hospital appointments and the constant risk of surgery postponements. But now he had a diagnosis, he was under consultant care and, most importantly, he could see a way ahead through these uncharted waters. He had been handed a lifeline. Hope. A reason to keep on living.

—

As if from nowhere, Tom found himself telling his two friends everything – about the job he hated, the physical and emotional toll of his health issues, his suicidal thoughts. Harri and Owen were soon sitting one either side of him, each with an arm around him like a rugby front row. He felt stupid, ashamed, embarrassed. He feared what else he might say. But he had no control. The alcohol, the emotions, the feelings took over. He told them how the pain had taken him to the very darkest places of his mind and, in those deepest moments of despair, how easy it would have been to take that step. To stop the pain forever.

The MVD procedure was a success. Five hours of neurosurgery identified the cause of the obstruction to the trigeminal nerve and released it. When Tom resurfaced from the anaesthetic, it felt like his head was going to explode and, even with his eyes closed, the light in the room burned through his eyelids and deep into his brain. Despite this post-operative trauma, the trigeminal neuralgia pain had disappeared with the surgeon's scalpel. In the days and weeks after the surgery he felt only tiredness. The physical pain was gone. And the suicidal thoughts? Gone too. As if they had never existed.

In fact, Tom didn't even register the disappearance of the mental and emotional anguish. Why would he? His voyage was complete and although it would take him a couple of months to fully recover, he slowly got his life back. Everything was neatly boxed away.

As he sat there, his friends' arms around him, he started to wonder why he had been so dramatic. Why had he opened this box? Was he attention-seeking? Was his life so shitty that he needed to put his emotions on display like this? Was he trying to be meaningful, relevant? Or was he actually broken? But he couldn't think straight. The sea wall had broken and as the water flooded out, his words mixed with his tears.

———

Tom lay on his back, his head thumping. He could feel every beat of his heart in his head. Was it blood pressure or a vacuum caused by dehydration? Either way, it hurt like hell and brought back bad memories of his life before the surgery. He was fully clothed in a sleeping bag and he suddenly felt very hot. His jeans were twisted around his legs, his upper body trapped inside his t-shirt and fleece. Sweat was beading on his forehead.

Eyes still closed, his brain registered brightness that baked his face and burned through his eyelids. He dared not open his eyes for fear of temporary blindness or worse. He had a flashback to a postoperative headache, light piercing through his eyelids, trying to split his head open. His mouth was dry and getting drier. He could hardly open it. The taste was horrendous. He could smell the alcohol on his own breath.

He remembered the food, the alcohol, the conversation. The conversation. Oh no. He felt disappointed with himself, ashamed, stupid... hungover to hell.

Now he became aware of the firm foam mattress and decided he must be in the forward cabin of *White Lady*. He remembered Owen designating him this billet the previous evening. He could hear a hushed conversation coming from the saloon and the aroma of fried bacon wafted in.

He slowly lifted his head, then his shoulder and upper body, until he managed to prop himself onto his elbows. At last, he opened his eyes. They were dry and sore and he was still wearing his contact lenses. No surprise there, given the state he was in. Today was going to be a long day, especially with the sailing they had planned. Before that, though, he would have to face his friends. The dread hit him like a dinghy boom and was quickly followed by a wave of sweaty nausea.

With a hollow bump, he swung his legs off the berth. The voices stopped. After what seemed like an eternity, Harri broke the silence.

"Are you alright, mate?"

Tom mustered a light-hearted reply, "I've felt better," lifting his aching, poisoned body slowly to protect himself from banging his head against the deck head.

He walked slowly into the highly varnished saloon. Owen and Harri were sitting where they had sat when the Radiohead track filled the air the night before. Had they been awake all night? Discussing him, analysing what he'd said into the early hours?

Deciding how best to handle their basket-case of a friend when he eventually emerged from the forward cabin?

The bacon and egg baps and the mugs of tea reminded Tom of their family camping trips. A vision flashed across his mind of the three of them sitting with their wives in fold-up chairs in a shady campsite near Hereford, drinking copious amounts of tea and coffee, joking and laughing about the fun they'd had the previous evening, while their children played nearby.

Now, with his head still pounding, he questioned why he had chosen to drink red wine last night. He'd discovered that alcohol – and red wine, particularly – rendered the medication ineffective. So, he'd quit drinking. So, why had he drunk so much last night? Was he trying to prove something to Owen and Harri? To himself?

—

Tom couldn't remember for sure what he'd said the night before. He didn't care. The door had opened for him to share his feelings. Now, in the clear light of day, he wanted to go over everything again. At that moment, he became self-aware. Aware that his friends were hanging on his every word, listening for the smallest change in tone or the slightest break in his voice. He told them about his journey, the days in the darkness of his mind, the emotional low points, the wanting to be dead, the not being able to talk about it to anyone. And wanting to stay 'strong' for the sake of Sarah and the boys.

He saw the pain in their faces, the shock, hopelessness, anger. They listened, asking occasional questions to help him get it all out. To his surprise, he no longer felt tearful. If anything, he started talking as if he were an authority, an expert on himself. He found he was able to articulate and externalise his thoughts and feelings without the noise of his mind, as he braided strands of sentences together like rope.

Harri and Owen had witnessed Tom's pain during a family camping trip near Builth Wells. Tom remembered that trip too. He had woken up early on the second morning and taken a sip of water from his plastic sports bottle. He was immediately hit by an electric shock that shot across the right side of his face from his ear through his cheekbone and jaw. The pain had caused his entire face and body to tense in agony. He remembered wailing with his mouth closed so as not to wake the children, tears of pain filling his eyes. Sarah woke, recognising the signs of his torture, although she had never seen him in this much pain.

The episode lasted for over twenty minutes. While the horrendous pain persisted, Tom got dressed and left the tent to go for a walk, trying to distract himself until the pain subsided. When he returned to the tents, Owen and Claire, Harri and Vicky were out of their tents, deeply concerned. They had known for some time that Tom's condition was bad but were shocked to see the physical effect it had on him.

The following day, he had been hit by several more attacks. Harri sat with him outside the campsite coffee shop as he tried not to scream in agony. He could still remember Harri's face, filled with sadness and frustration at not being able to help, feeling his friend's pain. Tom had come to know that look. He had seen it in Sarah's face far too often. It was one of the reasons he had considered, hundreds of times, taking his own life. The pain was bearable, just, but the hopelessness and guilt of the emotional pain that he and his condition were causing Sarah and the boys, as well as his parents, was unbearable. He had not wanted to be alive.

Now, sitting in *White Lady* with wash from passing pleasure craft causing the boat to sway gently, Owen's and Harri's faces reminded Tom of the pain his condition had inflicted on others. He got emotional, but he was not crying. He was angry that it had taken so long to diagnose, angry at the impact it had had on those around him, angry that it had pushed him to the brink of death. But this conversation was not all about Tom.

"Why didn't you tell us how you were feeling before your operation?" Harri asked. "And when those thoughts came back again? We could have helped you. We can help you."

Owen was just as upset as Harri; the looks on their faces were enough to tell Tom that the answers to these questions were important to them both.

"I don't know," he responded. "Maybe I was scared. Scared of what you would think of me. Maybe I didn't believe it myself. Maybe I thought I had everything under control, mentally and emotionally, and everything would fix itself once I'd had the operation. And it did...for a while. But then the job and that awful meeting with Steve and Pete, and those feelings all came flooding back."

After years of being submerged, the words now surfaced with ease.

Tom carried on, turning to Harri, "One thing I know, is that when I had that attack at Builth, when the tears were streaming down my face and I was in utter agony at that coffee shop, and hardly able to look at you through the blurry pain, I wanted to tell you."

Now, he looked at both of them, "I so wanted to let you know what I had been thinking, what I had considered doing and even how I had considered doing it. But I couldn't. I didn't want anybody else to have to go through it. To endure it."

He paused. "It felt like being in a fish tank looking out. I was frightened. The loneliness was unbearable. And honestly, I thought it was all over after the operation. But I hadn't properly dealt with it. The last few months have shown me that."

—

Hours went by before the three friends finally emerged onto the deck of *White Lady* to prepare for the shakedown sail. To celebrate the inaugural sailing trip, Harri gifted Owen a captain's cap he had found on an online joke shop. Tom and Harri donned their own joke sailor hats and all three enjoyed a good laugh as they motored from the pontoon to the lock gates. They drew some welcome attention from the many onlookers, including the harbour master. It was all a welcome relief after the intensity of the morning.

They hardly spoke for the rest of the afternoon, other than to communicate as needed to sail the yacht. As they glided across the bay, listening to the slap of the waves against the hull and the rustle of the wind through the sails, each was deep in his own thoughts, processing the morning-after-the-night-before. Each was trying, in his own way, to make sense of this situation.

The course of the weekend had changed. Tom had changed it and he could not get away from feeling guilty for hijacking Owen's plans. The rest of the afternoon passed in a blur of sails and sea. Harri went below to catch up on some sleep. Owen handed the helm to Tom so he could fettle around on deck. And Tom decided to do his best to be normal, helping Owen out as much as he could.

Back alongside the pontoon, they readied themselves for the walk up the hill to Penarth. At the restaurant, they ate and chatted easily after their successful afternoon on the water, consuming much less alcohol than the previous evening.

"Check us out," Owen joked. "Saturday night and we're struggling!"

The conversation was light. None of them wanted, nor felt the need, to revisit what had already been said. Owen and Harri, however, talked with Tom about how they might be able to help him find a new job or make introductions should he ever consider returning to working for himself again.

"I've never been very good at asking for help from others," Tom admitted, "even close friends like you two. But if you're happy to help, then I'd be very grateful."

He lifted his glass and they lifted theirs. The pint glasses chinked together.

"Anytime," Owen said. "We're here for you, mate."

—

Before leaving on Sunday morning, Harri gave Tom an almighty hug. Tom felt his friend's energy and love.

"Pass on my love to Sarah and the boys, and give me a call. Let's chat soon," Harri said before walking up the pontoon.

Tom and Owen watched him in silence as he drove out of the car park in his Range Rover. Owen was staying on board a while longer to complete a few more jobs. He and Tom chatted for a while, before it was Tom's turn to set out for home. Owen embraced Tom with the same physicality as Harri had.

"I mean it. We're here for you. But get some proper help. If not for you, do it for Sarah and the boys. Give them my love."

The marina was still bustling as Tom walked to his car, replaying the conversations, thoughts and feelings, and the pain, the fear, the friendship and the love. Poor mental health had never been something Tom had considered. Like many people, he believed it was something that other, weaker men experienced. Not him. Now, sitting in his car, the ignition keys on the dashboard, he held the steering wheel like the wheel on the bridge of his shipwrecked life lying on the ocean floor. He was overcome by the pressure on his beliefs, his thoughts and his feelings. He had been drowning. But now, looking upwards through the darkness from the deep-sea floor, pinned down by the weight of the salt water pushing down on him, he could see a small pool of light with blurry edges, flickering on what might just be the sun on the surface, occasional rays breaking through the darkness and falling on him. They were rays of hope. He was going to be alright.

As he sat there, the salt water started to burn his eyes and he squeezed them tight. Tears rolled down his cheeks like waves breaking on his face. His grip tightened on the steering wheel, as he lost control of his emotions. His shoulders and then his entire body began to shake. He cried and he cried.

Gerwyn Tumelty: www.coronprojects.co.uk

UNBLOCKING YOUR HIDDEN STORIES:

What parts can you relate to, about sharing with close friends?

How might your life change if you revealed your true self?

9

SHIFTING

Alison Westlake

When we read or hear stories that teach us something new or that resonate deeply because they remind us of something that has happened to us, it can shift our entire perspective. That shift can happen overnight or take more time. Some stories take time to filter through our minds, as we reflect, comprehend and apply what we have learned to our own lives.

Our lives thrive on connection, so our friends become the family we choose for ourselves. Although we love our blood relatives, the pressure of family can create different tensions in our lives. Life events and grief come to us all. If the trauma of an event is trapped in our bodies, it may show up in symptoms of pain or anxiety. We may need some physical work to shift our symptoms, such as Beth's release through dance in Growing. (Chapter 3)

When I met Alison Westlake, we talked about the power of massage as another way to help the body process trapped emotions. What I didn't know then was that she was also a therapeutic coach, giving her clients emotional support to complement the physical touch offered by healing massage. Here, she shares a story that reveals the power of working with the body.

Owning your Destiny

It was Thursday and I was off to my regular Pilates class. I had been going for a few weeks and was just getting to know the teacher and Pilates for the first time when the teacher told everyone in the class that I was a massage therapist. I blushed, feeling all eyes on me.

I was still a newbie in the group after all. I acknowledged Jane, a woman in her early fifties, on the mat next to mine.

The class began, with Jane occasionally turning to me to mouth, "I can't do that move." I could see the pain in her face as she gripped her right shoulder in exasperation. We chatted at the end of the class and Jane booked a massage session with me for the following week.

She arrived at my house in a chirpy mood. We chatted on our way through the kitchen to the garden and my therapy space. She fussed over Buster, our family dog, and asked, "Is he part of the therapy?"

"He is sometimes," I smiled.

"Why don't you start by telling me more about your typical day," I asked her, as the consultation began. "What kind of work do you do?"

She told me she worked in an NHS dispensary. "I've been doing my job for years," she said. The years of bending forward over the patients, years of care and commitment, showed in her body.

"Tell me about your arm," I said.

"It's so difficult to do this," Jane said, attempting to raise her arm above her head but wincing in pain before bringing it down sharply again. "I can't even dress myself. I feel like a 90-year-old."

Her frustration showed in her face. She was taking a range of medicines – amitriptyline, naproxen, escitalopram, antidepressants, HRT, multivitamins.

"I've got a headache today," she added, "and I'm fed up with not sleeping because of this shoulder pain." She recounted the past two years of increased pain and decreased mobility.

"What else is happening here?" I thought.

"I'm studying for a Master's degree, so I'm at a desk a lot of the time." I could sense that she was putting herself under a great deal of stress.

"Oh, and I've got pain in my thumb, from my shoulder down my arm," she added.

Now that I had this picture, I could plan a suitable massage. I told her I'd start with her back, shoulders and neck and then work on her pectoral area and along the clavicle.

As I navigated my way around her back and shoulders, I checked in, "How does this feel, Jane? Would you like more pressure?"

"Oh... no... that's lovely. It's hitting the spot," she mumbled from the massage table. I could feel her body desperately needed more care and a lot of work which I couldn't complete in one session.

Back in her clothes at the end of the session, I offered some feedback. I suggested a course of six weekly sessions to relieve her pain and get her shoulder mobile again. I explained how her being overwhelmed was stopping her muscles from working properly and they needed to be re-educated to switch on and off when needed.

"How does that sound to you?"

"It sounds like you know what you are talking about," Jane said. "My shoulder feels better already!" She paused for a moment, "Yes! I'm going to do this and get myself sorted!"

I sent her away with shoulder exercises to do each day.

"The exercises have helped lots," she said when she returned the next week for me to work on her relaxation and mobility. By the third session she had more range in her shoulder.

"I've reduced some of my pain killers," she told me. "I don't want to be on them and this is helping my shoulder so much." I was delighted to hear this. "Jane, that is amazing. Well done you for staying so positive."

But she was far from out of the woods. She arrived at the fourth session with a headache.

"It's all down here and across my shoulder," she said, as she touched her neck and shoulders. I focused the massage on those areas and gave her a head massage. She fell deep into relaxation.

The next week, Jane said that she had been doing well until two days earlier.

"My neck pain has come back. I think it's because of my sleeping position. We got a new bed because I wanted to improve my neck and back support. Seems like it's done the opposite!" she said in frustration.

Jane continued with her exercises and her range of arm movement continued to improve. But the pain shifted, giving her earache and causing her to grind her teeth. "I've had shooting pains down my arms. I thought I was getting better."

Jane's disappointment was palpable when she arrived for the sixth session. I suggested an oil blend to take home and use whenever she was in pain.

"It'll keep you going until I see you next," I offered.

After all the work we had done, I felt she needed something else to support her, especially now that she was no longer taking so many painkillers.

"I've been exercising more because my arm has been feeling better. But I think I must also know my limits."

"You're doing brilliantly," I told her. "But don't overdo it. Your body is still repairing and it's better to take baby steps."

"I know," Jane replied. "I also fell down the stairs last week and have some pain in my jaw and a bruise on my arm. It's keeping me awake at night."

"Is there anything else going on for you right now?" I asked her.

She explained that she had a Master's exam looming and was staying up late to prepare for it.

"It's how I've always done things," she said.

I suggested a gentle and relaxing session, with no thinking or talking, for her to 'just be' for an hour.

Spring 2023

By April, Jane's shoulder had improved and she continued to see me every month. Yet, in one session, everything had seized up with an unusual amount of tension. "Maybe it's the aftermath of your fall and the exam stress?" I suggested. Jane agreed.

However, I became increasingly concerned for her health over the following months.

"I seem to be suffering from tunnel vision and tingling in my arms and legs," she said. "It's lasting for twenty minutes and leaving me wiped out for the rest of the day. It could be hormonal. I'm still settling in with my menopause treatment."

Something wasn't right. "Have you been to the GP?" I asked.

"That's my next appointment," she said with concern in her voice.

I told her I would work with the acupressure points on her sacral area and shoulders to relieve a range of menopausal symptoms. While I could relieve a lot of the symptoms, this was one for the GP to diagnose.

Summer

Jane arrived the next time with 'niggly shoulders.'

"It might be hormonal," she said. "I was given a new desk at work. It didn't feel as if it was set up properly for me. I had to do a bit of negotiating, but I got my old desk back. It feels so much better."

I worked on the acupressure points on her feet to calm her mind, ease headaches, and help with irregular menstruation and irritability.

She was again experiencing residual shoulder pain that I was just managing to keep at bay.

"I've been doing a bit more with my family recently. Now the summer holidays are here, I've been cycling with my boys."

She sounded very positive that she was enjoying time with her family.

Autumn

After a summer break, Jane got back to her regular monthly sessions.

"I'm up to my neck with studying again, I was able to take a break from my Master's but I'm back at it again," she said. "I can feel it in my shoulders."

Her shoulders were generally much better these days and the range of movement had improved.

"I'm taking less medication now and I'm pleased about that," she said, with a small sense of achievement, "but I am still sitting at a laptop and writing a lot, at home and work."

Despite saying that she was feeling "chipper," she still had pins and needles down her arms and around her face. She was holding stress in her body from all the pressure she put herself under.

"When I get my Master's degree, I'll change my work," she said, "because I'll be able to work more flexibly in the private sector."

She seemed to be making the situation more pressurized by only seeing one path forwards.

Winter

Improvement to Jane's shoulder had slowed which could have been because our bodies don't heal as quickly while in hibernation mode. I suggested we try the AromaTouch Technique, using eight essential oils placed along the spine and feet and massaged into the back to reach homeostasis.

"I feel you need some rebalancing," I said.

The next session, she was feeling quite stressed, as I prepared to start the treatment.

"My husband is going overseas to visit his family and I'm still studying. I know he will be fine but I worry that he's going to a country at war."

I suggested a relaxation session focused on the head and shoulders.

While Jane's husband was away, she was feeling overwhelmed and looked exhausted.

"I'm running on adrenaline, and now the migraines are kicking in."

I focused on massage, stretching to release her tight neck and increasing her range of movement again, finishing the session with reflexology.

Spring 2024

Jane returned to her sessions.

"My husband is home, thank goodness. It's such a relief to have him around," she said.

She told me they'd taken up running together, but it was affecting her ankle. On top of that, she had to submit her dissertation in two weeks.

"I'm feeling good, considering the pressure," she said.

I feared that she would experience burnout when her levels of adrenaline dropped, once she turned in her dissertation. I suggested reflexology and found her adrenals were very enlarged and painful and her kidney reflex points were popping. Pressing on these points would bring relief, but the real medicine was figuring out why they were enlarged and then making the necessary lifestyle changes.

Thankfully, in the next session, she said, "I'm taking a brief break from studying now that I've finished my exams, I'm feeling exhausted from studying and life."

Summer

"Yes!! I've passed my Master's exams," Jane beamed, "and I'm very glad for that to be done, for now. Eleven months of hard work is finally over!"

I was delighted for her and asked how she was feeling.

"I've given myself a month off before I start my next Master's. I've been catching up with decluttering, gardening and the usual parenting responsibilities. I've also taken some medication for my headaches," she told me.

I felt there was something else she wasn't mentioning. "What do you think might be causing the headaches?" I asked.

"My father is in hospital," she said, "which is another stress. I've been busy visiting the hospital and running my mum around."

I worked longitudinally, to release her back and gluteal muscles and gave her a lovely head massage to destress and decompress.

She told me she had decided to cut sugar out of her diet. "It's helped me to feel less lethargic and have less of a fuzzy head," she said.

After the session she said, "I feel quite spaced out and like I've been able to release lots from my body." A positive result.

The next session, Jane was feeling anxious again and back on her meds because of work.

"I've started walking again though, because it seems to help me get things out of my system."

"Shall we focus on releasing the legs, feet and ankles?" I asked.

"Yes please," replied Jane gratefully.

And this time, she fell asleep, fully relaxed on my table.

Autumn

The children were back at school and Jane had begun a new Masters. The days were getting shorter and then the bomb dropped!

"I've been signed off work for two weeks with anxiety," Jane said with a sense of failure. "I'm sorry I'm so emotional. I can't talk to my mum at the moment. I will when I'm ready. My husband is very supportive. He's been helping with all the chores."

She reached for her tissues as she began to cry.

"I've been doing a lot of walking. I just find myself walking for miles and miles."

This concerned me greatly and I gently offered Jane the space to explore her reasons for walking, given her admission that her hamstrings and right foot were painful and she limped when she walked. Her knee was painful too. Everything on her body was aching and screaming at her for attention and self-care.

Today would be about holding space for her, with reflexology to calm and reduce tension and acupressure for her knee pain. She yelped when I applied the acupressure but, after a minute or two she said it was starting to feel better. I then massaged her quadriceps to release pain and tension from the front of her legs. She left the session feeling physically better but needing more time mentally and emotionally. I offered her a therapeutic coaching session for the following week.

We began the therapeutic coaching session with grounding and breathwork.

"I'm at crisis point. What do I do with that?" she asked, in tears.

"This is the point at which you cannot get any worse," I told her. "Now you can begin to move up and forward, albeit in small steps."

"I feel broken," she said. "There is so much for me to do. How am I going to do it all like this?" She began to cry more and described the feeling of anxiety rising in her body.

"My heart is racing, I feel so embarrassed."

I guided her through the session, providing her with the space she needed using her breath to calm her and connect with her somatic narrative.

"Oh, I feel so angry!" she cried out. "Angry with work and how much I've given of myself to my studying and to others. I've been back to the doctors and told them I need another month off. I think I need longer to get myself out of this situation."

Yes! Her resilience was starting to break through. She was starting to take back control of herself and what she wanted. I took her through some somatic work to help squash feelings of anger towards her job. This helped her to feel calmer.

She'd recently been able to share her experience with her Mum. She confessed that simple tasks, such as filling in forms at home had become too much for her.

"My mum has had to support me with this. I felt utterly out of control and helpless."

More somatic work helped her to acknowledge what was good in her life and her body, and helped her to listen to what her body was trying to tell her. This helped Jane to realize how disconnected she had become from her body.

"The signs were there before, but I didn't listen to them," she said. "I ignored them when I should have been prioritizing myself."

Jane now sought clarity about her next steps. She felt determination in her body and spoke about her goals and how she wanted her life to look and feel. We challenged the barriers to what might be holding her back and began to talk more rationally about her situation.

We gently discussed the steps needed to succeed. I could see a shift happening within her.

At our next session, she confessed that she hadn't done any of the grounding or breathwork exercises I had assigned her.

"That's okay," I reassured her. "Sometimes the deepest work is done when we listen to our body. Your body wasn't ready to move to the next step."

Jane had been through a year of stress that had impacted her body, mind and soul. The effects had led her to a crisis point. She needed much longer to rest and recuperate than she had initially realized before starting another new Master's in early autumn.

"I really can't do any research or continue with my studying right now," she said anxiously. "Even the thought of it makes me want to vomit. I want to make other plans. I have some ideas," she said with some hope.

In some ways, this way of thinking helped Jane to feel that she hadn't completely lost all hope. But she still had a great deal more self-healing to do. We paused a moment for somatic breathwork.

I asked her about returning to work.

"I'm not ready," she said emphatically. "There are lots of things that I've realised I'd love to do. I feel that I've missed out on so much with my family. I'm really struggling to juggle it all. My family means the world to me and that's all I want and need to focus on at this moment."

Gently we wove our way through the session.

My job was to stay on the riverbank, and never to jump in and save her. Jane had the answers within her; she just needed the time and support to find them. I set her the task of noticing more – of what was going on in her body and of being more connected with her mind and body. When she was more mindful of her body and mind, she had the power to set boundaries. Especially with herself. Jane left feeling much more empowered about her next steps and their importance to her.

At Jane's massage session a few days later, she said, "Last night I had no pain in my body, and I slept well. A call with my boss went well and I feel much better now. I was worried about what she might say but she was quite understanding, and I felt reassured."

"Would you like an AromaTouch Technique today?" I asked, intuitively feeling that this was what she needed.

"This session was the most relaxed I've felt in a very long time," she said afterwards.

"I've stopped my new Master's that I started in September," Jane told me. I could see the transformation in her.

Winter 2024

Jane continued to come for sessions. There was a new glow about her.

"I'm playing music in my house. It helps to lift my mood. I've never done that before. I'm more mindful now that my migraines are set off by stress. They're less frequent now and I've returned to work."

Spring 2025

Walking in, "I've decided to retire from work in two years' time!" Jane said, brimming with a new certainty.

"I didn't realize that I had to make changes in a different way for a better outcome. I've been stuck here for such a long time. Thankfully, you have helped me to reframe my way of thinking. What I thought was the best way to progress for my future retirement brought too much pressure for me to cope with. The years of being mentally, emotionally and physically engrossed in my work had all taken their toll. I have a plan and I'm still walking."

She sounded determined.

I smiled with pride and satisfaction for Jane, for her finding herself again. I can't wait to see what the future holds for her.

Author's end note: my work with massage for the body and therapeutic coaching for the mind shows how important it is to take a moment and breathe. To work out what we need for ourselves and who we can turn to for support. It can take a long time to reach self-awareness and more time to learn what our bodies are telling us. Life is for living, experiences, friends, laughter, joy, connection, support from and to others in equal measure. We are allowed to choose our own outcomes as well as help others. Be kind to yourself and find the spaces where you feel safe to listen to what your body is saying or even share your stories.

Alison Westlake: www.thehealingpath.uk

UNBLOCKING YOUR HIDDEN STORIES:

Which books that you've read have shifted your perspective?

How has exercise or relaxation helped you think more clearly?

10

LISTENING

Kimberley Vallis

We all know how it goes. When someone starts talking, it's hard not to jump in with an observation or a similar story of our own. Yet, the best listeners hang fire and let the speaker completely finish. Great listening builds an invisible bond of trust and intimacy, demonstrating the value the listener has placed on the speaker's words.

For the listener, a benefit of listening to stories is the slightly hypnotic effect of hearing someone else's voice. Observe what happens next time you are listening to an audiobook, or a speaker at an event telling a story. The brain focuses on the sound and gets busy making sense of the words, precluding all other thinking. The gentle rhythm of sentences calms our brain enough to bring us into a parasympathetic state. Listening to the pattern of a story gives our brains time to relax and move into the 'rest and digest' state, thus alleviating the stresses of the day. I have a friend who loves to chat on the phone while driving. It's no surprise that we often talk about the weather (yes, British!) because light-hearted, inconsequential conversations make us feel good. Whether we are children or adults, listening to stories has the same calming effect on us. In those calmer moments, we are better able to listen to the wisdom of our hearts and the instincts which our bodies hold. As explored in the last chapter, our bodies may be struggling with symptoms such as panic attacks, or stress-induced illnesses such as headaches, and then it's even more important to notice and listen to your body.

Kimberley Vallis is no stranger to the benefits of sound and the power of listening to your body. She began using singing bowls with her own children and then trained to be a sound therapist and practitioner. Listening to her own intuition and her family's needs became a turning point in her career. Her fictionalised story covers some of that journey.

Listening to your soul: A journey back to self

Frances 'Frankie' Vales had always done the 'right' thing. The right job. The right marriage. The right structure. But there comes a time in every life when 'right' begins to feel wrong, and the whisper of truth can no longer be ignored.

It began one grey morning when she felt an invisible weight pressing down on her chest. Panic. Stars sparkled and spun before her hazel eyes, her ears blocked as if they were underwater, sweat trickled down her temples, her vest top stuck to her back. In the past week, she had already endured two panic attacks, but this third one felt different. Not just fear. A reckoning. Her body was speaking what her soul had been whispering: something had to change. She sat upright, wiping away a flyaway strand of hair, reflecting back on what had happened over the last couple of weeks to lead to this moment; her terrifying fear in the dark...

Do the right thing, not the easy thing

Three weeks earlier, the night before her resignation, Frankie had a vivid dream. She was sitting obediently in the main hall of the school where she worked, the headteacher towering above her, pointing and laughing, while the rest of the staff watched on in silence. The dream felt painfully real. No one defended her and she felt shame, humiliation, sadness. When she awoke, heart racing, she dismissed it as anxiety. But the next day, it happened. The dream unfolded almost exactly as it had the night before, as though her subconscious had been preparing her, warning her.

During the first INSET day of the new year, the headteacher started running through the new rules and regulations for the school, and Frankie, as had happened in the dream, spoke up against the rules and how she would be expected to implement them.

"It doesn't sit right with me to take away the basic human rights of children and focus so heavily on attainment, rather than enlightening and inspiring their young minds. We are these children's and young people's guardians while they are here. We cannot take away their right to use the loo or to drink when thirsty. We shouldn't reprimand them when they are struggling. We cannot put our adult needs and wants, tracks and grades, over the well-being and safeguarding of the children in our care."

She was met with mostly annoyed silence, but also some tutting and eye rolling. The headteacher stepped up to the microphone on the podium. Her voice boomed about statistics, data, staff well-being, undermining everything Frankie had said about looking after, supporting and inspiring the young people in their care.

Frankie's face reddened. The sighs and eye rolls continued. When the tea-break finally arrived, Frankie marched to her classroom and sat at her laptop. Her hands trembled as she wrote her resignation letter and de-registered Harry, her eldest son, from the school at the same time. It was done. No turning back.

Back in the here and now, fear swallowed her whole. Hospitalised by another panic attack that this time felt more like a heart attack, she lay wondering if she'd broken everything. Her marriage, once solid, now felt strained by unspoken tensions, and a shift in roles and finances. All three of her children were now apparently home educated, without proper planning around how she and her husband Toby would pay the monthly bills. Her husband, while supportive, could not always understand the depth of her inner disquiet. But there were moments – tender, stolen – when he pulled her close in the quiet of night, whispered his faith and trust in her and in their marriage, touched her in ways that reminded her that she was still whole, still wanted, still wonderful. They made love not as routine, but as reassurance, as connection in chaos. These were the embers that kept them alight, that kept them fighting as a team and trusting in the process and the uneasy new journey ahead of them.

The household pulsed with challenges: Harry had complex sensory needs, Aiden was showing signs of emerging behavioural and sensory differences, and George was a toddler, needing constant attention. Chaos met uncertainty at every turn. To find time to even think about a new career seemed impossible.

Frankie prayed and spoke to the heavens – releasing all fear and surrendering to the serendipities and synchronicities that lay ahead. She slowed down. Breathed. Walked in nature. Journalled by candlelight. Attended sound baths where vibrations settled the storm within her.

She met kindred spirits in woodland forest groups – mothers, mentors, truth seekers. A local tribe of wellness and education renegades welcomed her in, keen to learn from her too.

As the noise of the old world faded, she heard a different voice – her own. Frankie took moments out to acknowledge how creative, dynamic and determined she was, spending natural unplugged time in woodlands and forests with herself and with her family, leaving behind the strained system of sleep, work, family, sleep, repeat.

She went from survival mode to LIVING mode. Putting a hand against her chest, over her heart space so she could feel her heartbeat and the warmth of her touch, she would sit and listen often to what her heart said.

During one sound bath meditation, listening to the chimes and soothing sounds, Frankie visualised a completely new path unfolding for her and for her family. The walls and barriers of her own life were gone. She was calm and connected with the job she needed to do... still teaching, still mentoring and still inspiring but with a focus on life skills, health and wellness, creativity and connection. She was floating. She was now on a sandy beach, making sand angels and listening to the waves roll in. Her breath mirrored the rhythm of her dreamy waves until she stirred and landed gently back into herself, keen to get the dream moving. She told the vision to her sound healing mentor, and she knew that this visualisation meant something.

Playing with waves

Five months later, and Frankie was taking a break from working for a friend who ran an alternative learning provision, her setting for children and young people who had been excluded. She was in green, lush Corfu, standing at the edge of the sea. The Aegean winds wrapped around her like silk, and she closed her eyes and heard it again – instinct. Clearer than ever. She would re-train. With the sun warming her back and waves tickling her feet, she made the decision to learn the art of sound healing and to complete the Forest School Leader training that she had started.

Within days of returning home, she found a teacher. Singing bowls sang to her from adverts and shop shelves, as though they had been waiting for her. She opened up, collecting a team of instruments and tenderly learning their ways, tones and melodies.

At the same time, she completed her forest school training and practiced gently with her own children, discovering the openness, freedom and joy that learning in nature could bring.

From this space of stillness, The Edventure Project was born.

Be the change

The idea had whispered to Frankie long before she left mainstream life. It was drawn in crayon, imagined in quiet moments. Now, the vision roared. Of a place where children could learn freely. Where their differences were strengths and not diagnoses. Where parents found solidarity and support. Where facilitators guided and mentored with compassion, not correction. Where everyone was happy.

Trusting her instincts again, Frankie reached out for someone to support her idea, to help her find the place and to make her vision a reality. And the Universe responded.

One sunny day, during a family picnic in a park, as the boys played in the sunshine, enjoying the space among other families and friends, Frankie sat on a checkered rug with Toby, chirping like a songbird about her incredible idea and how it would look, be and, most importantly, feel.

"We could do something really special. Make a real difference..."

She was cut off mid-sentence by a tennis ball landing on the rug.

Kayla, a wellness practitioner who had been playing catch with her daughter, had overheard what Frankie was saying and had missed the catch.

"Oh, my goodness," Kayla said. "I was just saying this the other day to my sisters. About how rubbish it all is and how my nephews are not thriving. I am worried about my son too."

With that, Kayla sat down. For the rest of the afternoon, she and Frankie connected, laughed and planned. It turned out to be such a small world – their husbands knew each other of old, and the two couples had shared friends and shared values. *Thank you, Universe*, Frankie whispered.

Together, Frankie and Kayla formed a community interest company and began building from the inside out. News of what they were up to spread locally. Frankie found the perfect place to set up the company but, when moving day arrived, they literally couldn't open the door.

"I can't open it," grunted Frankie as she shoved it with her shoulder. "It looks like it doesn't fit the frame."

"You're just doing it the wrong way!" Kayla hollered, dramatically miming giving the door a good yank with a wink and a grin.

However, no matter how they heaved and hoed, they realised that something was not right. Frankie called the landlord. When he turned up, they discovered a badly timed blip in their plan. The building frame certainly had moved and, along with it, the entire structure. The building was sinking into the ground beneath them.

Not to be deterred, the two dynamic and determined friends adapted, rented village halls and attempted to win over sceptical councils. Intuitively, Frankie knew the project was a wonderful opportunity to support families that didn't fit in the mainstream, rigid box, or that had slipped through the formal social, emotional and mental health net.

Families far and wide were keen to join the project, but not everything ran smoothly. Frankie's dream faced some resistance. The local parish council, unsure of what to make of this 'unusual' home education project, scrutinised the project and voiced their doubts. There were letters, meetings, and backhanded comments about legitimacy.

"What do you mean we cannot use a playing field to play in?" Frankie stood firm.

She showed the data, ticked the boxes, told the stories and never let any of them see her sweat. Beneath the surface, the panic stirred – but the old Frankie was gone. This time, she faced the veil and walked through it. With that, the magic began and the moments of serendipity became more pronounced and more obvious.

With pure abandon, Frankie began to trust the process in earnest. She multi-tasked her focus on Edventure and on her practice of wellness through sound. During one soothing sound session, a client approached her. Recognising Frankie's potential as a healer and master of the modality, the client suggested she train to become a Reiki practitioner.

Frankie put it to the universe and instantly found herself signed up for her first degree, serendipitously, with a friend she knew; a friend whose husband was an incredible builder and tradesman, with the tools and know-how to engineer a sinking building and to help it rise again.

Let's do this

The Edventure Project opened on Frankie's thirty-seventh birthday. It instantly became a sanctuary for the misunderstood, the charismatic and the clever. Children previously labelled as disruptive because of their behaviour or need, found rhythm in nature-based, hands-on learning. A boy once excluded for dysregulation became a dancer, his movements synchronised with joy. A lonely girl became a comedian, laughter echoing where silence had once reigned.

Frankie supported them, but it wasn't their stories she was living. It was hers.

Each morning, she arrived barefoot on the dewy grass, singing bowls and a coffee in hand, and strolled and breathed deeply of the earth and of her own power. She wasn't just leading others home. She had returned to herself. The Tribe, as she called them, supported each other and supported her.

Frankie's marriage transformed again. There were hard conversations, tricky moments of disconnection, but also rediscovery. Toby joined the project, saw her fire, touched her soul. Their reconnection and further alignment came slowly but grew with each passing day.

At the heart of it all was Frankie's unwavering trust in her instincts. She had risked comfort for calling, predictability for purpose. She stopped apologising for her sensitivity, for needing rest, for not fitting into tidy boxes. She began living from her centre – wild and wise and grounded. Through this exploration and this trust in her soul purpose, this really knowing and following her instincts, more magic flowed and unfolded.

Soon, Marla joined the mentoring team and the project's vibration raised again, this time, with a new creative spin!

Over the months that followed, Frankie and the Tribe awakened into their own power, as each of the young people and the mentors furthered their connections into themselves, overcoming the disempowerment of the labels that had been placed on them. Autism Spectrum Disorder, for instance, was transformed into Sensory Integration Spectrum (SIS), Deep Pattern Insight Profile (DPIP) and Authentic Communication Spectrum (ACS), leaving disorder and deficit in an outside world that failed to understand the needs and strengths of these young people.

With Frankie's guidance, Edventure grew in strength. The energy of the team grew and those who had been anxiously selectively mute found their voices through all forms of communication, singing and dancing, in front of audiences and, more importantly, in front of their families.

Entire families are able to breathe again.

Years pass. Frankie sits in a wooden hut filled with handmade treasures and art. Outside, animals stir and begin their day. She takes a deep grounding breath.

A robin comes to the door, singing its merry tune.

A new empowerment and wellness centre has just opened its doors, offering guidance and care to more families, creating more merriment and more laughter. Frankie exhales slowly. This was always the path. Not the easiest. But the truest.

In rising, she says, quietly, we lift others too. The robin replies with a knowing tune.

The Edventure continues.

Kimberley Vallis: www.theedventureproject.co.uk

UNBLOCKING YOUR HIDDEN STORIES:

What project have you been dreaming of recently?

Where in your life could deeper listening help you - are you hearing your own intuition?

11

BELONGING

Debs Penrice

Stories reach us on emotional and spiritual levels. When our imaginations are engaged with a story, our sense of belonging is supported. The human need to belong is one of our primary drivers, slightly higher on Maslow's hierarchy of needs and yet fundamental to our survival. If we don't belong to a tribe that can help us meet our physiological needs (find food, maintain shelter, sleep) and our safety needs (health, emotions, financial security), our nervous system stays in fight or flight mode. When that happens, underlying anxiety runs as a theme through all our behavioural responses, because our emotional brain takes over from our logical, reasoning prefrontal cortex. On the contrary, when we feel like we belong, it calms our nervous system, helping us to feel more supported, allowing our thinking to move back to the naturally positive intellectual brain.

One of the reasons we tell children stories is to help them understand the culture and tribe they belong to. The stories communicate ideas and goals to those younger generations, helping them decide how they want to live and what will help them fit in. However, some of these stories can perpetuate unrealistic expectations or negative opinions instead of bringing in positive expectations. Think of Disney: how realistic is it to expect the life of a princess or true love? Think of how witchcraft is represented: Are spiritual and magical skills always the work of darker forces? This short story explores a fantasy world of time travel, how it feels when we don't belong and the potential for us to communicate without words in the tribes where we belong.

The time-travelling telepath

Timeless space

She floats as an orb. A ball of energy. Thoughts flow to her and she lets them go. Some bring colours to her surface edges. Her energy burns a brilliant red as she sees a vision of a home – a roof and walls. Then her energy turns orange as she sees thin, pale leaves bound together. She tries to recall the name for this bound parchment, but the word escapes her. The first and last pieces are harder, protecting the thin sheets inside. These hard covers show images and undecipherable squiggles designed to protect what lies inside from all but the sacred knowers who can read them.

Next, a yellow-gold colour floods her energy. This is knowing itself. She has no word for it as it vibrates fast through her. Other energy orbs float around her and she can see that the nearest one is affected by her energy too, as it shimmers with the same colours in a different order. Flash. Her yellow turns green then flushes rapidly pink. The depth of colour feels like falling. She is drawn towards the other orb. Could they be closer? She floats. In that moment, the other orb explodes in the same colours as her – the deep green blushing to the pink. The colours match and magnetise.

All at once, the gap closes, each slamming into the other's energy. Softly landing. Then rapidly expanding. She feels herself growing, his thoughts now blending with hers. Their energy expands further, and she sees the brightest blue spread through his energy, instantly mirrored in her own field. There is no sound, but she feels the communication arrive in her consciousness,

We are one as masculine and feminine. Belonging. Our energy will grow and glow together, stronger, making us a beacon of light and healing in this universe. Our love reflected.

She doesn't understand all the words, but their sentiments warm and soothe her. She feels all-powerful, peaceful, loved. Her energy rests while the colours cycle through light blue, indigo, purple and white. Vision after vision. She sees further into the universe; her energy remains melded with his. As they drift, she knows they will take turns: each of them resting while the other works. Scanning the universe, sending out energy charges. Now it is her turn to nurture those souls and to work, while he cleanses and refreshes his energy. They continue to grow and expand together as they work and absorb the light.

> Pop <

Central America 1420s AD

She finds herself running. Dry skin and burning feet. No water to be seen anywhere. Dusty, arid mountains, steep slopes and broken dry plants. If she doesn't soon find food and water, she will fall and most certainly die. Her family is dead from the droughts already. But hope! In the distance, a figure crouches on the ground. She can make out reddened skin, a skirt fashioned of rags and feathers, and soft bark strips. The figure is much smaller than her.

She feels safe enough to slow down. She doesn't want to startle the crouched person but, as she creeps closer to the motionless figure, she hears the most beautiful sound. A song she recognises.

Her heart leaps at the notes. She needs to relearn that song, understand its lyrics, and make that sound. Suddenly, the figure stands, muscles stretching, bones cracking. An instruction which arrives as a thought in her mind without the strange woman even speaking,

Come with me. I will ask the chief if you can eat and stay with us. I am the shaman and you can learn my craft, if you wish?

She thinks of her reply, sending it with gratitude, *Thank you. I am Lee and I am curious how we can communicate without speech.*

The shaman smiles and holds out a hand for Lee's support. They walk together, past shelters and small dry huts dotted between the arid trees. They come to a tall man by a pool of water. He indicates that she should drink from the pool. His voice cracks open the silence,

"Welcome. Your true name is Liana. You can join our tribe only if you will accept me as your chief and keep the promise to learn our shaman's craft. You cannot leave us and you will find us again after each passing."

With a shiver, Liana acknowledges he has guessed her name correctly. "Yes, I'd love to stay."

"Good. There is much work to do and our shaman, Angelia, needs a healer to help her. I will pair you with a man to protect and work for you."

As if drawn by an invisible order from the chief, the men line up to greet her. As Liana walks down the row, feeling awkward and afraid that she doesn't belong, the chief and the shaman watch her. In the silence, before the chief can pick, a man steps forward, and Liana hears what can only be his voice in her head, *It's you. You're here.*

The man speaks, "It is me. I will do it. She belongs to no-one, but I will work for her."

Liana turns and looks into his piercing deep blue eyes, questioning, *Me?*

Out loud she asks, "For always? You'll be by my side while I learn the mystical path and work in gratitude for my keep and rescue? I would have died in the desert and I have no means to trade for food..."

> Pop <

Southern England 1660s AD

Her consciousness awakens more slowly this time. Pain, sadness. Her beloved brother and beautiful tiny mother are dying. She feels fear knotting her belly, stopping her from eating the last morsels. Her brother, her exact likeness, stares weakly back at her, his male form shrinking before her as the disease ravages through him. His dark red hair falls onto his oval face and into his green eyes, his chiselled nose dribbles. His wide smile vanished from his lips the day they heard of their father's death. Papa had gone to isolate himself once he could no longer work, but it hadn't saved the others. How could she bear losing her mother and her dear twin too?

They drift in and out of consciousness and she knows their end is close. Her heart aches as their thoughts collide in her mind. In an urgent mind-voice, Mother says, *When we pass, go to the workmen's lodgings and beg for work. You can serve. You are strong and quick. But do not let them see your mind-melding skills or healing touch. Simply cook and clean for them. Hide in plain sight.*

Her brother lovingly suggests, "Conceal your looks. Darken your red hair and dirty your face to protect your virtue until you find a safe home." Mother and brother pass within moments of each other. She has no time to mourn them.

She runs through the night, holding back her sobs. At dawn, she presents herself to the leader of the workmen's lodgings on the cliff top near the castle. She had seen the chalky cliffs stretching out along the sea and comforted herself with the thought that she could escape to swim in the sea as often as possible. Seeing her exhaustion, they give her a meal and a room.

The hours of work are long and harsh, but her daily swims restore her strength and endurance. As her brother had advised, she dirties her hair, ties it back, and hides her smile.

One day, a man comes to the kitchen, bleeding from a cut to his arm. She drops her book, which she isn't reading but rather using as an excuse to sit down; the squiggle letters are too difficult to understand. She enjoys the peace of sitting with it next to the warmth of the stove.

She rises from the floor and holds the man's arm, gently washing and binding the wound. She notices his bright blue eyes. Turning his head away from the wincing pain, he asks her gently,

"What book do you have? And who taught you to read it? Your father?"

She shakes her head. "I cannot read. I enjoy looking at the words, but none make sense."

He nods, "Would you like to learn with me, when I have time between my work shifts to teach you? I will collect you from the kitchen and we can find a grove where we can focus."

She finds herself smiling, knowing she can trust him. "Thank you."

She works faster each morning to clean the kitchen before his shift ends. They spend hours stretched out beneath the trees, as he works out how to teach her all the letters. One afternoon, she falls asleep mid-session. He realises she is exhausted all the time and sees that he cannot protect her from the harsh work. Another time in the kitchen, he hears another man insulting her simply because she is a servant and growing older with no prospects.

One autumn day, he plucks up the courage and asks her, "As one of the skilled carpenters, I have been given a hut of my own, so I can move out of the men's quarters and lead a team. That means I can marry. Will you have me?"

Her green eyes widen, her cheeks flush. "But you will lose all standing, taking an orphaned servant as a wife. Why would you do that?"

His tone grows quiet, so she has to lean in to hear him. "Because I care not. Anything to be in your presence, where I belong. It will be our home."

They are married in the tiny chapel above the castle, by a sympathetic priest who agrees to wed them in the absence of a witness. As the years pass, she bears him four bonnie children, all with her wild red curling hair and his bright, familiar blue eyes.

But her husband cannot keep her safe from the bullying attention of one of the men she had once served in the workhouse. He wonders if that man had known her father and bore a grudge. She bears the abuse well, hiding her bruises when he trips her in the market or tips her basket to the floor. Her loving smile stays bright but he watches her shrink and hide her truest nature.

Her husband is much older than she and begins to suffer the ailments of a body exhausted and wracked with disease. She curls around him at night, holding him close and sharing her healing energy. One terrible night, she realises he has passed. She cries out, "You cannot leave me here alone, my teacher, my only love."

As she drifts into dreams, she hears her family calling her home to escape her overwhelming grief.

> Pop <

Scotland 1790s AD

She is running again, this time in sturdy shoes down a filthy cobbled street, a basket of fruit and vegetables bouncing on her arm, threatening to spill its precious content. She has been spotted in the market square working her skills and is now forced to flee. With her mind-voice, she calls ahead to the young man, as he disappears out of sight beyond the next street.

My son, my love. I cannot go back. I must escape again. Otherwise, I will hang for my sins or burn for my witchcraft. This food must be delivered to your father's kitchen. Can you get it there safely?

Instantly, he responds in her mind, *Yes, Mother. I can take it from here. Meet me in the alleyway.*

She switches direction towards Squeeze Gut Alley, sending him her reply, *I'll be there, but it's not safe to linger. I cannot hope to hide my mind-melding thought-talk any longer so we must stay silent now.*

There he is, on the corner. Her son, with the most beautiful blue eyes and unusual red-blond hair.

She ruffles his curls and pulls him close for a hug, speaking out loud this time, "I must leave you. Your father is stern but fair, although you haven't seen him as often while he works. Go back to our home and he will teach you and keep you safe until you're old enough to join his company. Learn his master building craft if you wish but keep your mind-melding skills private, for he will not understand. I love you always."

"Thank you, Mother. I will not mention those skills of ours ever again. I love you too."

> Pop <

Germany 1990s AD

This time she is in a car. She sits bolt upright in a bid to stay awake while they drive for miles from Calais, up and across Belgium, crossing the border near Aachen. These days, she feels bereft. Sadness is close enough for tears to spill down her face whenever she is alone. She hates falling asleep at night because her dreams are wild stories, confusing images of lives and people she does not recognise. She searches, but for who or what, she does not know.

Eventually, the car pulls up to a large white, detached house with a tall metal blue gate. She grabs her only suitcase and her rucksack out of the boot, and steps up to ring the bell on the gate. She grips her luggage tightly, feeling like her whole life is packed into it.

"Guten Tag und willkommen bei uns hier in Wolfblasenstraße. Höffentlich hattest du eine schöne Reise hinein?"

The unfamiliar words overwhelm her. Yet, she translates, *Good day. And welcome to us here in Wolfblasen Street. Hopefully, you had a good journey?*

How will she survive a whole year here?

Her German is pretty good, yet it is strange to be here at last, hearing an authentic accent. She looks across to her parents, standing silently on the pavement. She will not be returning home with them. Her father chain-smoked for most of the drive from Calais, while her mother's silent anxiety brewed beneath her forced smile. She knows her mother tried to keep the conversation light but five hours in the close confines of the car had been torture.

Her parents will separate soon. They are selling the old farmhouse; their lives now packed away into boxes and suitcases. Her mother has shown her the secret bank account book. For every penny her father has spent on tobacco, her mother has squirrelled the equivalent away for a rainy day, saving up for when she needs it most. She knows she will never step inside her childhood home again. She turns away from her parents to focus on the present. She smiles warmly at the frazzled woman standing by the gate, then follows her up the path to the front door. Children appear down the stairs and from the garden, and the woman calls the youngest two to her side.

"This is Maximillian. He is two, nearly three. And Betsy is four, starting kindergarten in September. Peter is six and Katrin is eight, almost nine. Katrin, Bitte Schatz, will you show Leanne her bedroom and bathroom?"

"Danke sehr Katrin," she says in her faltering German, as she turns up the stairs to follow Katrin.

The bedroom is large and airy, painted white with two pictures on the wall and a homemade sign on the door bearing her name. She sinks down onto the narrow single bed, lifting her feet and staring at each wall in turn to get a feeling of the space. She wants to stretch out under the duvet and cry. Instead, she stands up and returns downstairs to say goodbye to her parents. She finds them having a drink with her Hausmutter, but soon they will be on their way. She guesses it might be hard for them to leave her in a foreign country just days before her 18th birthday. But her mother has insisted there is nothing to hang around at home for, so they celebrated her birthday a week early.

The next morning, her Hausmutter says, "For your birthday, we'll go to the Circus am Rhein and see a fortune teller."

She understands and is curious. She's never had a psychic reading before. She settles in and learns more about her job and the children's routines.

On the day of her birthday, they set off with Maximillian on reins, Betsy holding her hand, and Katrin and Peter running ahead and circling back to their mother. Herding the children towards the red striped circus tents dotted along the river bank, she finds her stomach fluttering and a rush of tingling energy down her arm.

Her Hausmutter introduces herself to the woman in the tiny gypsy wagon, then ushers Leanne through to the chair and table, saying, "I'll take the children to the playground. We'll come back soon – enjoy yourself."

Enjoy myself? How? she thinks, twisting awkwardly in her seat as the mystic sits down opposite.

"You will find him but not recognise him, maybe he is a divine feminine this time?" the mystic begins, in heavily accented English.

"Always as one, he will teach you patience, joy and how to handle grief and rage. He will show you the deepest friendship and love but you will have to leave him. You are promised to another in this lifetime, for you have made vows to bear these special children. Check the Book of Souls when you find it, maybe you can find a way to unravel those bargains of chastity, silence, separation and obedience? Maybe they cannot be broken? Let us explore a past life and find another story which may inform your journey."

Relaxing her shoulders, she settles into the chair and grounds her feet to the floor. She imagines drifting, wandering, as she listens to the mystic's gentle instructions.

"Do not attach any emotion but let your mind float effortlessly through time and space. What can you see? Where are you and what kind of ground are you on? What is your form and what are you wearing? What do your eyes see and how are you feeling?"

Half an hour later, Leanne emerges into the sunlight from the darkness of the gypsy wagon. She throws herself on the grass, pulls her notebook from her bag and hastily scribbles down every detail.

She remembers being a strange tall form, wearing long white robes, working with crystal balls and great glass telescopes. She watched bright energy orbs become human lives and she read and documented human stories in far-off lands. Her male colleague, working alongside her, wore the same robes. She watched his brown eyes stare thoughtfully through the observation window, the feelings, colours and energy shifting as the stories unfolded.

He smiled at her, encouraging her to face the truth. "After years of watching, it's nearly our turn to join them. Is your story ready? What will unfold?"

In that moment, the form in white robes realised her energy was twice its natural size. In the same second she made this discovery, her masculine energy separated itself from her heart, unwinding into its separate physical form.

She sighed, "I know we have to go separately."

Her heart ached as her other half moved away, still staring back at her with familiar blue eyes.

Leanne stares at her notes, not really understanding what they say about the masculine and feminine energies. Slowly, she gathers her things and goes to meet the children and their mother to return home. Together with her Hausmutter, they feed the children tea and birthday cake, before she races for the 7pm tram. Today is her birthday, after all. After such a weird day, she can't wait for a pint, and her new friend, Sasha, another local au pair, is meeting her for a meal before they start celebrating.

Full of pizza, she and Sasha laugh as they run down the steps into the Irish bar.

"We can speak English all night here," Sasha shouts over the din, promptly pushing her way into a crowd of hellos.

These were Sasha's crowd of friends, random people she has met over a year that is about to come to an end as she prepares to return to the UK and university. Sasha boldly pushes Leanne forwards, telling everyone they are celebrating her birthday and her arrival in the city.

Suddenly feeling shy, she looks across the group and briefly catches the eye of a tall, dark-haired man as he lifts a pint to his lips. The next moment, she is rooted to the ground, giggling helplessly as the girl with bright blue eyes next to her cracks another joke. She glances across at the tall man again but then turns back to Sasha and the laughing girl.

The strange boyish-looking girl with blonde-red hair triggers a sensation that feels like heartache and a long-buried memory as Leanne looks directly into those bright blue eyes. The girl's lips don't move, but Leanne is sure she hears the girl's voice in her head. *You're here.*

Yes, I'm here, she silently replies and sees a small smile of acknowledgment on the girl's face.

Out loud, the girl invites her, "Hey, it's *my* birthday in two weeks. Why don't you come to my house party to celebrate again?"

Debs Penrice: www.storyhealing.net

Unblocking your hidden stories:

Which places have given you the greatest sense of belonging in your life?

What experiences might you write about if you were tasked with helping someone else feel less alone?

12

Reflecting

Richard Sutcliffe

By the time we reach 40 or 50 years of age, life has dealt us many different cards. Maybe we've experienced partnership and a breakup or three. We might have become a parent or aunt or uncle, and now have small people in our world. Maybe we've moved location and re-built our home or completely changed our career. Perhaps we've faced the grief of loss. We each have so many different stories to reflect on, some of which are explored by the contributors to this book. Yet, no matter what the story, they all have one thing in common: other people and our relationships with them. Even in our professional lives, how we relate to our bosses, colleagues and clients often drives the emotional undercurrents flowing beneath our busy lives. All the time, our brains are checking in, first asking 'Am I safe?' Then, 'Do I belong, am I loved?' And, finally, 'Do I have purpose and meaning in the world?'

When we face difficulties, it is the love and support of the people around us that gets us through, and for some people, their spiritual faith. Most of us find that telling a personal story and feeling listened to are cathartic for the soul. This is what Richard Sutcliffe found when he worked on *Finding Mac*, his memoir about becoming a father. What he wrote about much less was the journey of 'finding Richard,' some of which he charts in this fictionalised story about the life of a rather jaded village priest, who listens to others in his role as a different kind of father. His reflections reveal that all the people we meet in our lives have a purpose for us, reflecting back on us the very things we need to notice, learn, embody or appreciate in life. They are all parts of our story.

Confession Saturday

It was the most glorious sunny day in Longwall St Jerome (or simply Longwall to the locals). One of those warm, early summer days when the air was completely still, clear and fresh, with a deep blue sky. Richard remembered how his dad always referred to this colour sky as Carolina blue. There was a light breeze but in the sheltered spots, you immediately felt the warm sun on your skin and could almost imagine Vitamin D being made by your skin. This was normally the sort of day that Richard loved – but not today. Today was the first Saturday of the month and, as was tradition, he would be hearing confessions at Longwall's Church of St Gerard. It was the opportunity for the local faithful to unburden their souls to Richard, enabling them to sin without worry for another month, in the sure knowledge that they would receive absolution next time. *That's a pretty uncharitable way to think of things*, Richard thought. He often found confession to be a trial in itself – the same people trotting along each month. They always shared the same list of fairly mediocre and trivial sins. On the very rare occasion that a parishioner revealed something juicier, the seal of the confessional meant that Richard couldn't even share it with anyone.

You see, the truth was that Richard didn't think of himself as a particularly good priest. He was good enough at all of the set pieces – Sunday services, baptisms, weddings, funerals – but when it came to the personal and the pastoral, he wasn't really sure he had the patience for it. In many ways, life had left him jaded. Things that would have excited him and felt important when he was younger and more naïve and eager, just seemed to bore him now.

It wasn't even as if confession was really much of a thing in the Church of England. But here, in this rural corner of Hampshire, formal confession had stubbornly hung on, probably only because the Church of St Gerard had one of the finest examples of a confessional booth in all of England. It had been installed by Reverend Canon Leo St John-Smythe, a former rector of the parish, in the late 1800s as part of the Anglo-Catholic revival. The beautifully carved mahogany structure had been designed with a door leading to either side of the confessional – one for the priest and one for the penitent – and a grille separating the two, which retained, in theory, some anonymity for the latter. The worst thing about the booth was the seat. Sat there for several hours, Richard found the wooden bench rather uncomfortable for his increasingly ample backside. A range of cushions, brought from home, helped to make things a little more bearable. Yet another reason to loathe this particular Saturday.

With all these negative thoughts running through his mind on this beautiful morning, Richard opened up the church, went to the vestry to make a cup of much needed coffee from his secret stash of 'proper coffee' (and not the unpleasant brown sludge the church wardens insisted on serving after the Sunday service) and went into his side of the confessional. He adjusted his cushions, said a prayer as he placed the purple stole over his shoulders, and waited for the first penitent.

Reflected love

The usual suspects had gathered and were ready to unburden themselves. First, as always, was the trio of Hannah, Josephine and Jessie – widows of a certain age and stalwarts of St Gerard's. The three raced to the church on each first Saturday, each keen to be the first to tell all their sins to Richard, as if unburdening was a highly competitive sport. Month after month, they said the same stuff, inevitably leaving Richard bored stupid. He found himself going through the motions, merely replying without any real thought.

Hannah was first today. She prattled on, then began to talk about how she missed her late husband. Howard, who had died five years earlier, had been a wonderful man, a stalwart of the village, always ready to help those in need. Goodness shone from him and he was missed by everyone. What Hannah really needed from the confession was an excuse to talk about him. And as she talked, Richard drifted away to thoughts of Swee...

He'd had lots of friends when he was young, but romantic relationships never seemed to work out for him. More often than not he found himself safely in the 'friend-zone' – always available for advice and a shoulder to cry on, but never much more.

For as long as he could remember, he had wanted to be a husband and a father. There was something innate in him that responded to taking on that special responsibility. Even when marriage and family were far from the thoughts and desires of his peers, they seemed the natural order of things for Richard. As he got older, he began to accept that maybe it was never going to happen for him. Having plans was fine, he decided, as long as you could accept that you would need to alter them as circumstances changed.

When he bought his first house – a two-up, two-down Victorian terrace in South Wimbledon, complete with polished wooden floors and pretty fireplaces, he wanted to stamp his mark on it. He asked his sister, Sandra, and her oldest childhood friend, Swee, to help him decorate it. Swee was very artistic and relished the opportunity to use her skills on the house. Richard and Swee had known each other for most of their lives. They shared a sense of humour and increasingly, over the months of planning and carrying out the redecoration, spent more time together, often meeting up or just chatting on the phone and invariably laughing at something very silly. Looking back, you might say they were (prepare for a very old-fashioned term) 'courting'! But neither was ready to admit that. Their friendship was too important to risk.

On the next Valentine's Day, Richard received a card. Although Swee had only plucked up the courage to send it anonymously, Richard was pretty sure he knew who it was from. That was all that was needed for the pair to make the leap. What followed was the quickest of engagements, and a wedding in December of that year.

They enjoyed a very happy married life, despite having to negotiate a few 'bumps in the road,' as most married couples do. Somehow, Richard and Swee were just better together. He was the louder, more extrovert one; she was quieter but, deep down, much more daring and willing to take risks. He tended to worry more, but her quiet, unfailing support gave him the confidence to push forward with things that he might otherwise have found too difficult.

The first significant 'bump in the road' had been when they tried to start a family. After a year of trying and monthly disappointment, they embarked on the brutal journey of IVF. Hormones and emotions hammered Swee's body and mind at every stage of a process that was ultimately unsuccessful. The final route open to them for parenthood was adoption. After a lengthy process, they welcomed Mac into their lives. Richard was now the husband and father he'd long dreamed of becoming.

Now, vaguely listening to Hannah's ramblings, Richard thought of Swee's face. Although not conventionally pretty, her face shone with love. He had always believed that you could see the truth of someone in their face. Real love and genuine care for others shone in peoples' faces. The love they had was reflected in the light that shone out of them.

The Transfiguration – in which Jesus is seen to glow on the mountain while appearing with Moses and Elijah – was one of Richard's favourite Bible stories. It reflected his belief that the more you loved yourself and others, the more the love of God shone through. He had seen that most in Swee, who reminded him of a line from *Les Misérables*, one of their favourite musicals:

"To love another person is to see the face of God."

Richard, pulled back into the present, realised that he was talking to Hannah about Howard. "He was such a warm person, Hannah. Love shone through from him – it always does. And I promise it does from you, too."

He shared the quote with her. "You have nothing to confess today. Continue to go out and to love. Reflect your love and the love you shared with Howard in everything you do. That is the best way to honour him."

With this benediction ringing in her ears, Hannah trotted off, her next stop the local village shop where she volunteered serving tea and cakes, and sharing the glow of reflected love that she felt when she remembered Howard.

Reflected fatherhood

Richard got through Josephine's and Jessie's confessions, and a few others besides, but his love of coffee meant he soon had a full bladder, making him pop to the loo a bit too often. Thank goodness the church council had agreed to install a toilet five years ago. Before that, he'd had to take surreptitious comfort breaks behind an isolated gravestone – never an easy manoeuvre in a cassock!

After making yet another coffee and raiding the secret stash of chocolate biscuits (just for the energy boost, you understand), Richard reluctantly returned to the confessional. He saw Phoebe kneeling in the pew, waiting her turn. He took a deep breath.

Phoebe was a young mum whose husband, Rafe, was "something big in the city," meaning he was rarely at home. Phoebe had given up her own successful career to raise their four beautiful, but rather precocious children. Despite having enough money for as much help as she could ever need, Phoebe had wanted so much to be a mum that she was determined to do it all herself. After an initial struggle to get pregnant, many miscarriages and much prayer, Phoebe and Rafe's first child had been born six years ago. This first one somehow kickstarted Phoebe and Rafe into fertility, and they were now the proud parents of four children under six.

It's fair to say that Phoebe found Confession Saturday a welcome opportunity for a break from the children, who were left at home with their father! Rafe made sure that his mother and sister popped round on the first Saturday of each month to help with his childcare duties while Phoebe unburdened her soul.

Richard would have been more than happy for Phoebe to just have a doze in the confessional! She, however, relished the chance to speak to an adult and not to engage in baby talk for half an hour. Phoebe started to recount the latest mischief that her four 'little devils' had unleashed that week. As ever, Phoebe was feeling wholly inadequate.

Again, Richard found himself drifting off…

As it happened, Swee and Richard had always had adoption in the back of their minds as a route to creating a family. Richard's mum was adopted, and she was a good and successful example of how it could work.

They went along to a presentation on adoption in a random village hall somewhere in Hampshire. After this, they filled out lots of long forms and the approval process got underway. It wasn't easy. They were both told they would have to lose a large amount of weight before the process could even start, otherwise they would not be considered. So, they proceeded to lose several stones each. Over the next nine months, and after many meetings with social workers who looked at every aspect of their lives together, Richard and Swee attended a panel to seek approval.

They were finally given approval, but that didn't make the process any more straightforward. They drew on their reserves as they waited patiently for news.

Just as they had begun to give up hope that they would ever be matched with a child, Mac came along. For so many reasons, the match was perfect. On 14 November 2008, Mac moved in and they became a family of three – the little family Richard had always dreamed of.

Sitting in the confessional, Richard reflected on all those family times they had together. The holidays – especially those special ones in America with his wider family; Saturday morning drives to swimming and Tae Kwon Do lessons; playing silly water games on sunny days in the garden; building snowmen and having snowball fights in the winter until they couldn't feel their hands anymore.

During the adoption process, Richard had thought a great deal about what he would like his child to call him. Would an older adopted child want to call him 'Dad'? After all, that child would likely have, and remember, someone else in their life called Dad. The child's experience of a father figure might not be a positive one. He kidded himself that he wouldn't mind what he was called, but that was a lie. He was desperate to be a father and to have someone bless him with that name.

Of course, most adopted children are just as desperate to call someone Dad, so as soon as he moved in, 8-year-old Mac called Richard 'Dad.' He remembered the feeling of joy and fulfilment the first time and it was something he never took for granted.

Reflecting on his own past, Richard now found he was talking to Phoebe:

"The concept of parenthood is so important in Christianity. Our concept of God as Father, as a parent, is key to our understanding of that part of the Holy Trinity. When I was younger, I felt it easier to relate to God as Son, as human and walking alongside us. Now, as I have experienced fatherhood, it has given me a better understanding of our relationship with God as Father, as a parent.

"I understand more the intimacy of being one of God's adopted children. I understand more his desire to protect us and love us. I also understand more his need to let us go and to let us make our own decisions. I understand his desire and need to give us freedom of choice.

"Being a parent is hard, Phoebe, but you are doing a great job. Don't ever doubt that, and don't ever hesitate to ask for help. What I can tell you is that I have learned so much more from being a father to Mac, than he ever learned from me!"

Thanking Richard, Phoebe left the confessional, to return to her chaotic and busy life, but with the pressure lifted a little by his thoughtful words, just enough to get her through to their next encounter in a month's time.

Reflected loss

There was a lull around 1pm, with no more penitents waiting in the pews. At this time on each first Saturday, Richard normally had about half an hour to refresh himself, have a quick bite to eat, and get ready for the afternoon punters. The parishioners of Longwall St Jerome were a predictable bunch. Some confessors always came in the afternoon, having completed their household chores in the morning. Confession, for them, was a little break between the hoovering, tidying and dusting.

Richard had bought a rather nice pork pie from the shop, made with local pork and onion chutney. It tasted very good. He accompanied it with a quick gin and tonic from the secret bottles he kept in the side of the confessional. He wasn't sure what Archdeacon Hattie or Bishop Erica would think, but since neither really ever visited this remote corner of their patch, he didn't worry about it too much. He gave a wry smile.

The afternoon wore on, with more of the usual Confession Saturday penitents showing up to unburden themselves. But by mid-afternoon, the pew was empty. Richard was about to call it a day when he heard the familiar sounds of someone shuffling into the confessional and taking their place on the kneeler. There was a strong small of expensive after-shave – Richard recognised it as Jean-Paul Gaultier – and a voice he did not immediately recognise:

"Forgive me Father, for I have sinned, it's been ten years since my last confession. I just felt I had to come and talk to someone about this. The guilt is beginning to eat me up."

This wasn't what Richard was expecting. It was unheard of for anyone on Longwall St Jerome to confess anything of any real substance. He wasn't sure he was going to know how to help.

He replied, "Just tell me the story. Tell me what is troubling you so much..."

Hesitantly, the man began to tell his story. He recounted driving to work early one morning. The local country roads were quiet.

He wasn't really paying attention. There was a sickening thud, as something hit the car...

In that moment, Richard was abruptly carried straight back to the day he tried not to remember. He was instantly there, on 14 October 2016, with a policeman knocking at the front door.

This was the moment that Richard's life changed to 'Life after Mac,' the moment Richard learned that Mac had been knocked off his motorbike by a lone van driver and killed. It was a moment Richard chose not to think about too often. To be fair, it was a moment at once seared in his memory and which, in many ways, he could barely remember. It often felt as if he was watching someone else's life on a TV screen. But it had happened. It was real life. Mac had died just a month or so after his sixteenth birthday.

This really was the ultimate 'bump in the road' – the one that no parent ever wants to think about and certainly not something it was possible to prepare for. The next days, months and years were unimaginably difficult for Richard and Swee. How were they to find a way to move forward and be happy again? Was it even right to consider moving forward? What was their 'purpose' now that their longed-for and prayed-for child was dead?

They found things to do. In Mac's memory, they organised a sponsored walk and a night of music from the musicals, raising a significant amount of money for Children in Need. Most importantly, their loss drew Richard and Swee closer together, rather than driving them apart.

But Swee never got over losing Mac. She became more and more sedentary and rarely left the house. She mourned physically, with one illness after another as she became increasingly unwell. Suddenly, on 18 September 2020, a day before her sixtieth birthday, she collapsed and died.

And with that, Richard was on his own again, looking for a way to move forward. Once again, it was time to draw on a deeper well of resilience and find a new plan for his future. Often, when people heard his history, they'd say they couldn't understand how he could move past so much loss; or they'd tell him how brave he was; or they'd say it wasn't fair. The truth was, Richard had no choice. He could either move forward and live his life, or not.

On the day that Mac died, he made two promises – that he would not become angry and that he would find a way to live his life, as Mac, and now Swee, no longer could.

Richard found himself back in the present, sitting rather uncomfortably in the confessional on his improvised pile of cushions, listening. At that moment, he realised he did recognise the voice on the other side of the grille. It was George, one of Mac's oldest friends. The after-shave had such a familiar smell because both Mac and George had loved it.

Richard felt a pang of loss for his boy.

"George, I recognise your voice, my boy. You have never come here to confession before."

"Father, I just feel dreadful. When I hit and killed the deer, I felt so guilty. Partly, it was because I had hurt this beautiful animal, but mostly it was because, when Mac died, I promised that I would always take care on the road. What if it wasn't a deer that I had hit? How could I be so thoughtless?"

Richard was overcome by a wave of sympathy and affection. George had been a good boy. He had been a good friend to Mac, when others were still getting used to this newcomer to Longwall Primary School. He had put up with Mac's anger and bad behaviour when others had not been so patient. Now a man in his twenties, Richard realised how much Mac's loss had hit George.

"George, thank you for coming to see me, but please let go of your guilt. As we grow, we learn from our mistakes, and you have learned from this one. One thing I have learned as I have reflected on difficult times in my life, is that we need to learn from the past and not hold onto it. George, you get to live your life in a way that Mac can't. Living your life as the good and caring man that you are is your way to honour your friendship and his memory. He would be proud of the man you have become. I know I am."

With that, George suddenly burst out of his side of the confessional and in through the priest's door, giving Richard a huge bear hug; one of those hugs that reminded Richard so much of Mac and made him miss him just that little bit more.

"I was so worried about what you would think if I drove so badly. I was worried what Mac would think. Thank you."

With one last hug, George turned and left, seeming to skip down the aisle, leaving Richard quietly contemplating the day. He had heard his last confession for the day, so he returned to the vestry and quietly packed up.

As he walked home in the fresh, early summer evening air, Richard congratulated himself on getting through another Confession Saturday, not really sure why this odd tradition still endured at St Gerard's in Longwall St Jerome.

But his parishioners knew the reason. It was because of Richard! Despite his sometimes grumpy and curmudgeonly countenance, the villagers of Longwall loved him and valued his advice. Despite his dislike of the practice of formal confession, he always managed to find the right words, his love of his congregation and his love of God glowing out from him and reflected in him... even when he was feeling grumpy. He always seemed to find reflections in his own life that brought forth words of wisdom to those in need.

The truth was, Confession Saturday was here to stay!

Reverend Richard Sutcliffe:
www.findingmaccouk.wordpress.com

UNBLOCKING YOUR HIDDEN STORIES:

How does this story link to your own experiences of 'finding' yourself?

If everyone in your life offers a mirror reflecting something of yourself, what is it that you see reflected back at you?

13

Inspiring

Abigail Barnes

You know those stories full of adventure and bravery, and clever and complex characters? They inspire us. They draw us in with their energy, compelling us to make changes in our own lives. When a story lands like that, the impact may happen instantly or it might unfold in waves. Those heroes from stories and our role models in life are the people who inspire us. For some of us, characters in books offer that inspiration. It was the unstoppable nature of Jo in *Little Women* for me. She was fierce, yet soft and emotional, a walking contradiction. When an author creates a character that we can relate to and empathise with, it can profoundly move us. We might receive flashes of self-awareness as we compare ourselves to them or insights for what and who we want to be in future. One of the stories here in this book could inspire you to think about who would be interested in hearing your story. Perhaps it will inspire the next generation or someone who needs to know that they are not alone?

Yet like Kate/Katherine in Abigail Barnes's story, it may take months or years to figure out your story or to figure out the meaning of a huge life event. I got to know Abigail when we were introduced to talk about marketing strategies. We soon started talking about our love of books and their potential to change lives. And as I talked about some of the authors I had worked with, Abigail realised that fiction can be a great vehicle to release the last fragments of fear from a story, reveal the deeper message and truly inspire others.

Finding your purpose from trauma

Alarms are evil, Kate fumed, as she groggily hit snooze again, knowing it was going to be a rush to be first at work today. For weeks, she'd been struggling with motivation – not that anyone could tell because she was a world class faker. But life just seemed pointless.

Smiling, fawning, appeasing, placating; if they gave out awards for people pleasing, her name would be at the top of the list. She knew exactly how to act to navigate life – what to say, how to say it and, most importantly, how to dress for the part. It was no wonder she was struggling with motivation; she had no idea who she was any more and why she was even here. Not in a suicidal way but in a 'when is this chameleon life ever going to end' sort of a way. Would it ever be safe for her to simply be herself?

The alarm went off again, reminding her of what mattered and why – the buzz she got from being first in the office; how organised and on top of things it made her look to everyone that mattered. Perception was reality in her line of work; a lesson she'd learned the hard way.

On paper, her life looked good. She had a high paying job in financial services marketing, weekend trips to the south of France, a shoe collection to die for, a monogrammed Louis Vuitton Neverfull and a brand-new Prada handbag. But nothing filled the empty feeling that followed her around like a cloud. It was like she was stuck on a constant merry-go-round searching for something new to make her feel better; an aching hole that everyone around her seemed to be able to fill with parties, Prada, prosecco, promotions and pay rises.

There's a saying, falsely attributed to Einstein, that goes, "The definition of insanity is doing the same thing over and over, and expecting a different result." If it was true, then she must be insane, because she'd been trying all those things for years to no avail. Heaving herself out of bed, she jumped into the shower before it had a chance to warm up, instantly regretting her mistaken conviction that cold water could somehow miraculously wash her low mood away.

With her fourteen-hour work days, she didn't have much time for a social life, or for sleeping for that matter – she was lucky if she managed four or five hours a night. She could never shake the feeling that she was living the wrong life. Every day was a struggle, and she knew her negative mindset, habits and actions were contributing to keeping her stuck. But she didn't know what else to do.

On the one occasion that she'd let her guard down and told someone how she was feeling, they'd looked at her like she was crazy, insisted she have another drink and then proceeded to tell her that booking an expensive holiday would make everything better and give her something to look forward to.

She followed the cold shower with a hasty black coffee, she had no time for breakfast and soon she was out the door, and on her way to work. At 11am, her boss called her into his office and told her he was sending her on her first overseas work trip. She was to go to Boston for five days of meetings. Kate realised that if she flew out on the Friday evening, she could spend the weekend with her friend, Sarah, an ex-colleague from a previous job who now worked in New York. Sarah was originally from Boston, so they could stay with her family and catch up while exploring the city.

For the first time in what seemed like years, Kate was excited. Finally, she had a purpose, her hard work had paid off, she'd 'made it' and her friend Sarah would, no doubt, have some sage advice for her too. She'd really missed Sarah's calming presence since she'd moved to New York a year ago.

In the run up to the trip, Kate felt stressed, pulling even longer hours than usual, desperate for everything to be perfect and for the senior colleagues she was trying to impress to be pleased with her. She reminded herself that she could sleep when she was dead and jokily told anyone who would listen that this job was killing her. It was a badge of honour to be busy. In her world, busy people were important people.

Three nights before boarding her transatlantic flight, Kate was forced to go to bed early. She couldn't stop the world from spinning or the black and white lights from flashing in front of her eyes. She was annoyed by this inconvenience. She'd never had a migraine before and didn't have time for one now.

Apart from that, and almost fainting on the train on her commute to work the day before she was due to fly out, she was in reasonably good health. Overworked, under-slept, living on snacks and coffee, like everyone else. But she was young. Her body could handle it. She'd decided to wear work attire on the flight, because that's what her colleagues did. Plus, she'd booked an evening flight which meant she could do a full day's work in London and arrive in the US in time for dinner, thanks to the time difference. She'd bought a new black fitted trouser suit, along with some white shirts and co-ordinating tops for the trip to really look the part of an international professional.

In her careful planning, she hadn't factored in that she would be eating an evening meal with Sarah's family at 2am UK time following an eight-hour flight. But hey, she was a business traveller now. She had to do whatever it took!

Flying business class was everything she'd dreamed of and more. The lounge was heaven, filled with every convenience imaginable, unlimited food, snacks and drinks, important looking professionals – and she was one of them!

Marco, the flight attendant, stowed her coat and made sure her champagne was topped up throughout the flight. He even fetched an extra bottle from first class when business class ran out. She was celebrating, she was excited, she'd made it. Finally, her life was turning a corner and things were looking up!

Sarah was at the airport to meet Kate. The two friends were excited to see each other after a year apart. They drove directly to Sarah's parents' house, where a warm welcome, delicious dinner and more wine on top of the inflight champagne awaited.

Kate fell into bed, drunk and jetlagged.

She felt terrible when she woke up the next morning and quickly started to feel progressively worse. This was different to any hangover she'd had before. The black and white lights were back. She was burning up.

Sarah's fast-thinking mum called an ambulance and her dad had to physically hold Kate up so that she could throw up in a dustbin as paralysis took over her limbs.

As the ambulance arrived, Kate's world slowed. Sounds blurred. She lay paralysed on the bed in the foetal position, terrified as she struggled to breathe and rode continuous waves of nausea and pain. Was she going to die?

Was this the end?

Suddenly she left her body and found herself rushing down a long dark tunnel and hitting a door at the other end. Where was she?

Was this death's door?

If so, it wasn't opening. That must be a good thing, right? She didn't want to die. Not like this. Not in a city far from home. Not at the age of thirty-two. Not with a life barely lived. Not in her pyjamas. Not in her friend's parents' guest bedroom!

She started begging – silently, maybe out loud, she wasn't sure – begging for more time, begging for a second chance, begging for help. Despite the lack of motivation and pointlessness she'd been feeling recently, she knew she wasn't yet ready to leave.

And then she found herself somewhere else. Somewhere white and vast. It felt like a waiting room and she could hear voices.

"She had her chance and she blew it," one said.

"But what if this at last is her wake-up call?" asked another.

"This moment has been a lifetime in the making," said a third. "It would be a shame to waste the opportunity if she could take it now."

Slowly it dawned on her. She must be in limbo, in the space between worlds.

They were talking about her, debating the pros and cons of giving her a second chance at life. The conversation sounded heated, like a case being tried in court. Only, who was representing her? And would she get a say?

Everything around her became distant. She felt as if she was standing on the edge of something vast and irreversible. This was it. She was going to die. In that moment, everything made sense. She wasn't ready. She hadn't truly lived. She had been waiting – for permission, for the right time, for the feeling that she was finally 'ready' to start her life. And now here she was, feeling that it might be over before it had really begun.

Suddenly, she was back in her body again, being poked and prodded, scanned and assessed. She was in the hospital. She was still alive and the medical team was hunting for a diagnosis.

Kate didn't remember much between the moment everything went black and when she opened her eyes again. It felt like a blank space in time, as if life had paused and then restarted. The first thing she remembered was the cold. Hospitals are always cold, but this one felt colder than usual. Artificial cold. She could hear the distant hum of machines; the quiet rhythmic beep of TV medical dramas. Except now it was real. It was hers.

The room was bright, like an interrogation room with every light turned up to full beam. Her mouth was dry and her head ached with the worst pain she had ever experienced. It felt as if her brain was too big for her head. She had a strange sensation of being aware of her body and checking it for damage. Could she move her fingers? Yes. Toes? Yes.

But everything felt slow. Like she was in a vacuum.

She turned her head slightly and saw a nurse adjusting something near the IV stand. Hours passed. She was moved to another hospital that had an MRI scanner because Sarah's dad had advocated for this.

Her physical body was in 3D, being looked after by the medical team, but her soul was on trial in 5D, and all she could do was let the waves of regret and realisation wash over her.

Finally, it all made sense.

The emptiness that had been her constant companion, the feeling that time was running out, the need to seek external approval and validation, had all been trying to teach her something, inviting her to question, to rise up, to become the version of herself who knew the universal truth. But at that moment, she lacked the consciousness to understand any of this.

She'd been trapped in a self-defeating victim loop, telling herself the same stories over and over, drinking away her misery. She'd been playing out patterns learned from others, living her life from their beliefs and getting similar results.

Fitting in.

A lifetime later (24 hours), Kate was woken up by a doctor with the results of the tests they'd carried out.

"You've had a stroke," he said.

Letting his words sink in, two thoughts immediately crashed into her mind. First, she was thirty-two years old and she'd had a stroke. WTAF? And second, she was thirty-two years old, she'd had a stroke, but she hadn't died, so there was only one thing she could do.

"Can I go to work tomorrow?" she asked.

This was a mess, but it was fixable. She was alive, so that meant she still had a job to do, and her boss would kill her if she didn't go to the meetings she'd been flown over here to attend. The show had to go on, the show always had to go on!

"No ma'am," the doctor replied, "You're going to the intensive care unit so we can figure out why this happened and to prevent further complications."

This sobered Kate.

The next seven days went by in a blur. The swelling of her brain subsided, the battery of tests revealed the stroke she'd had was a vertebral artery dissection (VAD) and not, as the doctor put it, "something more serious," and Kate found herself being discharged and ready to fly home.

The business class flight home was markedly different to the flight out. Her parents were with her this time, having flown to be at her bedside the moment the news of her hospitalisation reached them. The black business suit was replaced by a tracksuit and all she wanted to do was sleep. There was no Marco, no champagne and no idea what would happen next.

Kate would always be grateful that she walked away from her stroke without any physical disabilities. If you met her today, you wouldn't know she'd ever had a stroke. The PTSD from the event was manageable and most days the stroke was a memory for her.

But it happened. And it gave her a second chance.

She would never forget that feeling, that cold, stark realisation that life can end in an instant and you only regret the things you didn't do. That was the moment that everything started to change.

From that day on, things that used to matter no longer did. Things that other people cared about no longer seemed important. Kate was grateful for the second chance she had been given but had no idea what she was going to do with it and, some days, that felt more like a responsibility than a gift.

She never felt more alone than in the months after the stroke. No one seemed to understand what she was going through. She looked fine, so everyone wanted her to be fine. They wanted things to go back to normal, for her to go back to work and for her life to carry on. But she couldn't, because she wasn't the same person. Yes, she looked the same and sounded the same, but she wasn't the same. Kate died that day, on 25 February 2012.

It was Katherine who was given a second chance, a mission, a life purpose. But who exactly was Katherine and how on earth was she supposed to find her purpose in life?

For months, she went through the motions. She attended counselling, spent time with friends and family, laughed, smiled and spoke with gratitude. But most of the time she felt paranoid, lost and afraid, and not quite sure what she was afraid of.

All she knew was that the more people needed her to have a plan, the more tired and overwhelmed she felt. She was scared to leave the house, scared to make a decision, scared to speak to people in case they realised how 'crazy' she was.

Being such a young stroke survivor, there weren't many people she could speak to about how she felt. She couldn't join a group because she didn't have a disability, and she thought everyone would think she was a fraud. There were no books she could read or stories she could resonate with online. The counsellors she spoke to were appointed by her employers, so she felt it was better not to talk to them about how she was really feeling.

She had no idea who she was or what she was going to do next. And she had no idea how to fit in the way everyone else needed her to. Eventually, she was rehabilitated back to work on reduced hours, but it quickly became obvious that she didn't fit in there anymore.

Back then, personal development wasn't a mainstream thing but, one day, when doing an internet search for how to stop feeling depressed, she came across an American man who wrote books and made CDs about that very topic.

Those books and CDs became part of Katherine's everyday life and when his participation in a live three-day event in London later that year was announced, she booked a ticket.

On the day of the event, she grabbed a seat close to the stage. But in real life, this guy was huge and loud and wanted everyone to hug the person next to them and high-five strangers. She felt like a deer in headlights. This simply wasn't for her. At the end of the session, she felt deflated, in shock. The feelings she'd been hoping to feel didn't come, the next steps didn't appear. She'd been given a second chance, and she still didn't know what to do with it.

When he finished, she slipped out of the room and skipped the next couple of sessions, feeling like a ship lost at sea, with no direction, wind or crew. What was she going to do now?

On the following Monday, she was due to return to full working hours. She had been so sure that this event and this man would provide her with the answers and the escape she needed. She studied the event programme as she ate lunch.

The session after lunch was about how to become a paid public speaker. Not knowing what else to do, she returned to the auditorium and this time, chose a seat towards the back of the room. This speaker was funny and confident, with a four-step process that sounded easy to follow. Maybe this is what she was meant to do next?

Suddenly, he moved to the middle of the stage, walked slowly to the front, leaned forward and said in a stage whisper,

"Why do you try so hard to fit in, when you're born to stand out?"

An electric shock shot up her spine. He seemed to be speaking directly to her. Now she was on the edge of her seat. That's it, she heard a voice whisper in her ear, you're going to become a paid public speaker. The speaker announced a three-day speaker training programme that would take place in a month's time, near Heathrow.

She knew what to do next. She was going to become a public speaker and tell her story about how she had survived a near death experience. With her second chance, she was going to motivate people! And she was going to get paid to live a life of meaning and inspire others to do the same.

But just as quickly as she heard that first voice, she heard another, sneering loud and clear, *Who do you think you are? No one will want to hear you speak. You get nervous in team meetings. You'll never be able to do it.*

The voice had a point. She did feel self-conscious in team meetings. Besides, what did she know about running a business?

That night, she slept fitfully and attended the next two days of the event, mostly because she didn't have any other plans. On the final morning, she passed the public speaker's stand on her way into the auditorium. As she figured out what she would say to the man who had inspired her two days earlier, a woman appeared.

"Hello, I'm Dede," she said, with a friendly smile. "How can I help you?"

Katherine told her that she wanted to attend the three-day event near Heathrow.

She had a question that she felt was too silly to ask: *Could someone like her do something like this?* But she didn't ask it. It sounded as though she was asking permission. Not needing to ask permission was the first of many lessons she learned on the other side of life after near death as she began her journey into a new career and a new way of being. In the end, she completed the public speaker course and followed it with two others – one in internet marketing and the other in becoming a self-published author.

When people talked about becoming, Katherine envisioned it as being something like school. You sit in a classroom and someone tells you how it could be, teaches you the new skills and a few years later, off you go. You start your new 'entrepreneur job' with your new skills and live happily ever after!

She soon discovered it was nothing like that. Rather, becoming was like riding a roller coaster in the dark. One minute, everything made sense and, the next, she was feeling every emotion under the sun – imposter syndrome screaming at her 24/7, fear and uncertainty her constant companions and feedback from others her guiding light. This made for a difficult journey when these different emotions conflicted.

But if it were easy, everyone would do it.

A little over a year after her stroke, she said goodbye to her corporate career and became an author, a public speaker and a full-time entrepreneur. She'd never felt more alive. She'd also never felt more uncertain of who she was without her Blackberry, her business cards, her job title and her guaranteed monthly income.

Over the next few years, she invested in coaches, trainers, mentors and travelled around the world, slowly building her own training business, consulting with entrepreneurs and professionals, speaking at conferences and events, and writing books that shared her near death message with the world.

She learned from those hours spent in limbo in the hospital that no one is getting out of this life alive. Her vision asked her to let her life be her legacy, to live as courageously and intuitively as she could and to remind others that it's their time too. Even now, there are some days when the task she set herself can seem scary, as the things the vision asked her to do are often far outside her comfort zone. But, as one of her mentors often reminded her, something is not faith until it looks as if it might not work out but you still believe!

Trust the process. It's your time.

Abigail Barnes: www.abigailbarnes.com

UNBLOCKING YOUR HIDDEN STORIES:

Who or what has inspired you most in your life?

What would you do differently in your life today, if there were no consequences and no time limits?

14

REMEMBERING

Debs Penrice

As we get older, we carry greater responsibilities, making life feel more serious. When we are anxious, tired or overstretched, our feelings and thoughts fall into more negative patterns, as our emotional brain scans for potential dangers nearby. The voice of our inner critic turns its daily observations into judgements and makes up fear-based stories. We forget our usual positivity, and our behaviour starts to change. Stories and anecdotes can make us laugh and help revive our spirit, restoring us to our natural, lighter self. Being joyful and taking intentionally positive actions replenishes our energy. Being creative and tapping into our skills reminds us of who we are.

This is why solution-focused therapy approaches can help us to shift our perspective, look at who we want our future selves to be, making the best of our strengths, our values and the things we love about ourselves. The work in solution-focused sessions helps us to practice the skill of finding solutions, of finding those things that will make us feel better and of taking action. Our feelings follow the action. We shouldn't wait until we feel better before we act. We must do the thing now, even if it's a small thing. Finding peace in accepting self, returning to our joy and still learning new things can happen at any age. I've seen this with wonderful clients, even in their seventies. I wrote this story of freedom and remembering to honour the changes we can make, at any age in life.

Freedom from the inner critic

Judy

Oh, my goodness! My hair is such a state. It's not too far up the road from the bus stop but already the rain is soaking me through and my leg aches more when it's raining. This useless leg. So stupid of me to trip over and fall. I guess I'm too old to expect it to heal easily. I hope the trek over here is worth it. I wonder if this woman can really help me. She seemed nice on the call and seems to know her stuff.... But why did I agree to this? Therapy has never worked before... and what am I letting myself in for, with hypnosis? Surely, it's a stage trick. And she's thirty years younger than me. How can she possibly know what it's like to watch your kids grow into adults, your health get worse, and then find life so empty, feeling so disconnected from your kids and grandchildren?

Debs

Her knock on the front door startles me. It is 13:53. I'm not quite ready. Releasing a deliberately slow, gentle exhale, I turn on the speaker and tap the Bluetooth on my phone to connect it. A brief mental checklist, *Music, glass of water, box of tissues, session report sheet, blank paper, colouring pens.* Then I smile to myself and go to welcome the lovely Judy in. We have only met once, online, for her initial appointment.

"Hello. I'm so sorry, I'm a bit early!"

She breezes in, smiling back at me, a little windswept. As I show her in and where to sit down, I notice she's bursting to talk. She tells me she's spent the week at home, organising her spare room and sorting through some older clothes while preparing for her operation.

"I'm nearly ready for my friend to come and stay, but I'm worried she's going to be exhausted if I need more than just meals while I recover. So, I'd like it all clean and organised."

I nod. "Sounds like you've been working through it. What else has been good?"

"My granddaughter's got me into Vinted, so I could post up a few things on there. I'm not sure how well any of my old tat will sell, but I really need to make a bit more space, ready to move once my leg's better. My wardrobe is really overflowing."

I smile.

My own mum was always clearing out and frequently mentioned not wanting to leave too much stuff for us to sort out. Yet, the underlying energy was obvious to me: my mother didn't want her things to become a burden to us as she aged towards her eighties. But maybe it's something different for Judy? Only patience will tell me.

"You're making more space and planning for your house move? Tell me more."

"I love my place but, lately, it feels too big. I don't need all the furniture. And it's an old house that needs a lot of maintenance. I want somewhere smaller, where I'm not always calling Luke to help. He's a wonderful son-in-law, a wonderful husband to my daughter, Emily. But he's got such a busy job."

"He sounds lovely. And what if he enjoys that role of helping you? Maybe helping you is another way that he supports Emily? Our primitive brains lead us to think certain ways – perhaps more negatively, if we're feeling emotional. But we never truly know someone else's thought process or perceptions, unless we clarify it with them."

"Yes, I guess if he had no time free or didn't want to help, he'd say no."

"Hmmm. I think he would, if he's a busy guy. Perhaps you could ask him, next time you're feeling unsure? What else has been good in the last week?"

Judy settles into her seat and goes through some of the small things in her week that made her smile. She worries about Emily, who has a lot going on with two teenage, nearly grown-up kids. But she reminded herself that she had asked some gentle questions to open up a conversation with Emily and support her. And Judy had enjoyed shopping this week because she found the perfect present for her grandson's birthday.

"He was my first-born grandchild and, although I want to spoil my granddaughter too, it's his turn. Since he moved out, I see that he's becoming such a lovely, kind young man. But his love of Lego has never faded, so I found a Ferrari kit for him."

"Ah, that sounds like a perfect choice for him to relax and enjoy some quiet time. What else has gone well this week?"

"Well, I navigated quite a tricky situation with one of my friends. She wanted me to help with her evening fundraiser in a few weeks' time. But I'm already volunteering once a week in the charity shop. I love being there and interacting with people. And her event will be high stress. I don't mind going along to it. However, I don't want to take on a load of extra jobs until I'm walking more normally."

"So, tell me more about your leg?"

Judy tells me that she'd taken a nasty fall the year before. Walking the streets with her daughter to see the local Christmas lights on their way to the pub, she had fallen headfirst onto the pavement. The shock numbed the pain for a while; however, she now needed an operation to fix her leg because it hadn't healed properly.

"And how is it now?"

"I'm still waiting for the operation, but it's much better. I've been up to the park several times this week and I can cope with my limp. I can tell when I'm overtired though, because it gets worse again."

"It sounds like you understand how far you can stretch yourself, though?"

"Yes. But sometimes I can't help but get anxious about tripping again. And it spoils my time in the fresh air."

"You've got the operation booked now and hopefully you'll heal completely afterwards. What else have you been up to, to support yourself and prepare?"

"Well, I bought myself some sunflowers. I love them, so cheery in the sunlight or even on a grey day."

"Mmm. It has rained a lot lately. How has that affected you?"

"Not too much. I went antiques shopping with my brother when I visited him. Such a surprise: I've already sold one of the things I bought – for a profit. I love the buzz of the auction and I got some beautiful things."

"That's great news to get involved in something that interests you – when's your next auction visit?"

"Not sure yet, but I'll definitely go again. It reminds me of my career days in sales and merchandising. When I worked for a drinks company, I was even distributing cider – visiting all the pubs in the region."

"It sounds like you really enjoyed your career. So Vinted and the auctions let you have a bit of fun with buying and selling again."

"Yes, I guess so." She smiles back at me.

Eyes sparkling, she talks a little more, reminiscing about her busy days on the shop floor and then on the road in sales, and the wonderful and fun people she met. But soon her thoughts turn back to her daughter. I can see her compassion and how important being a mother was to her because, like so many mums, she had given up work for a while when Emily was young.

"We had lunch together this week and it was so lovely to see her taking a break instead of working the whole time. I understand that she wants to keep busy now the kids are growing up, but she seems exhausted."

Emily works in a law firm in the centre of Bristol. Even though her commute is fairly short, she often works until after 9pm. When she finishes in the office, she takes her laptop home for the evening and continues working after she's had dinner with Luke and their daughter.

I smile as I remind Judy that perhaps Emily needs her mum to show up in the city every so often, to help her take that much-needed break from the office.

"Yes, I guess we all need some help to focus on ourselves from time to time."

"Exactly. Small acts of self-care."

That reminds me to take a drink of water while we talk some more.

Judy

She's so understanding and so extremely positive... bloody hell. It's impossible to feel discontented or unhappy sat in the room with her listening to me. But what I'm saying is so trivial, what must she think of me? I get what she's saying about self-care, but it's always made me feel just selfish... I have far too much time alone and am always thinking of myself as it is. Surely my role is to help and support Emily and the others... I ought to be doing more, not less. But Emily's always been so capable and so different to me... she doesn't seem to need me... and it's just so frustrating that my leg isn't better yet... stupid old woman, tripping over like that.

Debs

I gently explain how our brain's reticular activating system focuses on gathering evidence for what we tell it to notice. So, when we ask it to be aware of all the good things in our week and all the small things that we are grateful for, it starts a flow of noticing more good things. But when we criticise or berate ourselves, those negative things seem to crop up more often.

"Have you ever spotted that happening...when one good thing leads onto another...and another? Perhaps it's not that the difficult challenges have stopped happening; rather, that they take up less space in your mind. Because you are busy focusing on the positives.

"And on that, how are you feeling this week, if you use our happiness scale from one to ten?"

"Probably a five. I'm excited about the auctions, but I'm feeling really lonely this week. Seeing Emily was great, but I haven't done enough socialising with my own friends since this leg."

"And if there was something you could change in the coming week, what would that be? What would help you climb back up to a six out of ten?"

"I'd take the bus and visit a friend who lives over by the university. She's got a lovely apartment, and we could walk in the gardens and go to the restaurant there, rather than sit indoors."

"So, what's the first step? Perhaps you'll make the call to your friend and suggest it? When might you get time to do that?"

"Soon. I think maybe Wednesday? Yes, Wednesday, before I go for my shift at the shop."

"How would you feel if you achieved that?"

"Really pleased. It'll do me good to get out more."

"Right, let's take some time for you to relax and let your mind drift for a while. Get comfortable on the couch and I'll pop the music on."

Half an hour later, Judy wakes gently from her trance state and sits up on the couch.

"Well done."

Judy smiles back at me and takes a deep drink of water before heading off for the week.

Judy

Oh, I feel lighter, more relaxed and a little more bouncy for sure. Did I fall asleep? How embarrassing. But I think I heard everything she said, loved the story about the little pebble... and that amazing colour yellow, so sunny and warm... it felt like pure love and connection. I feel like I slept... so relaxed... and my leg isn't hurting when I walk... that's better... like it is first thing in the mornings when I've slept well... that's a bonus! Perhaps I'll write some of the good things down this week...

Debs

The following Monday, Judy checks in and says how delighted she is that she's been to see her friend. They'd swapped stories of times gone by; the contrast of working and eating in fancy restaurants, then having toddlers and catering to their every demand for snacks and food.

"Funny, but I was remembering how much I hated to cook before I had Emily. By building up some simple recipes – not all of which she would eat, mind you – I became quite resourceful at managing our food shop funds. I enjoyed eating more veg and simple things. So, we got by and went on a few more outings."

"And how might that be useful now?"

"It's not the same cooking for one. I guess I could invite friends over for dinner a bit more often though. That would be fun."

"Mmm. Sounds like a great idea. What else has been good for you this week?"

"It sounds silly, but I found some new music that I like on Spotify. Have you heard of CMAT?"

"Yes, the Irish singer...?"

"That's her. I've been listening to her music and that led me to find a whole bunch more that I like. You know how Spotify makes suggestions?"

"Yes. It's good to listen and find new songs to enjoy, isn't it?"

"I think I'd like to go to a concert again when my leg is better, or do they call it a gig these days?"

"That's another good idea. What else have you enjoyed this week?"

Judy

I wish I had my notebook with me... I knew she'd ask me what's been good but now that I'm trying to remember, my mind's gone blank. Such a rubbish memory... And I meant to write them down... Silly woman... No, correct that Judy, that wasn't kind. Perhaps I could read my notes before my appointment next week? And, at least I have slept a bit better this week, so I can think straight if I just pause... and breathe...

Debs

I notice that Judy has stopped talking and I wonder if her worries are circling or if her memory bank needs a pause. I smile gently again.

"I'm worried about my energy levels. There are all these things I used to enjoy that I've stopped doing. It's too much in one day, if I've volunteered in the shop or been to see Emily."

"That's okay. Remember, the more we try and think about or do in a day, the more our bodies suffer from decision fatigue. So, could you make plans early, do one or two things and then relax for the remainder of the day and enjoy a rest?"

"Yes, I guess that's what I have been doing. It's just so frustrating."

"It does sound like frustration, but also, you're doing a lot to help others which takes a lot of energy. In this space, we are working together on picking the small things that you can control and enjoy entirely, and that don't depend on others."

"Yes... and there have been lots of little things. I've got a bench in my garden, and I've been taking a cuppa outside to sit there even in the briefest glimpse of sunshine, which has been lovely."

"Great. That sounds beautiful, if you can breathe in the fresh air without worries circling. Our state of mind improves when we take positive actions, or arrange positive interactions with the people who help us feel good. Those positive thoughts will help you to focus on believing that you will get better."

"Yes. And I called another friend who lives in New Zealand. We haven't seen each other for a few years but we always laugh so much when we catch up."

"So, how are you feeling, if I asked you to score your happiness out of ten this week?"

"Definitely better. Maybe a six and a half?"

"Great. And if I asked you to practise feeling a seven or more, what might you notice about your week? What else can you see yourself doing?"

"I'd actually sit down and read a book, instead of collapsing on the sofa and scrolling on my phone when I'm tired."

"So, when might you find time to do that? Which day?"

"Tuesday. But I think I'll save it for the afternoon."

"What time on Tuesday afternoon? Let's get specific and then your brain will hear you committing to the plan."

"I'll take a rest after I get in – about 4.30pm. I'll light a scented candle, make a cuppa and actually sit down for once."

"That sounds great. So, if you do that at 4.30pm on Tuesday afternoon, how will you be feeling?"

"Great, really pleased with myself."

"Time to lay back and relax for a little while, while we clear some of the things that were getting in the way of you making definite plans."

Judy sits up at the end of the session, drinks her water quietly and smiles at me.

"Thank you, see you next week."

Judy

Oh gosh, maybe I fell asleep again... but that's okay... it's good... Of course I can take an hour out... That sounds lovely and I will enjoy that new paperback. I'm looking forward to tomorrow now. Get a few chores done in the morning, head out but then rest when I get back. Sounds like a lovely day... I'll do it and, if the sun's shining in the morning, I'll get a cuppa outside and even pull up a few weeds.

Debs

Judy quietly arrives on time this week and I instinctively look for signs of fatigue or worry. There are none. She breaks into a beautiful smile, not forced; she seems confident and relaxed.

"Ah, it's so lovely to be here and you look so well too. It's been good to get some sunshine this week, hasn't it?"

She peels her jacket off, which I take and hang up.

"Yes, it's been so warm until today. Lovely, would you like a glass of water or do you need anything else before we start?"

"No, I'm all good."

"Well, funny you should say that – you look good – your hair's different. What's been going well this week?"

"Most things... everything... I feel like I'm back. I know I've got the operation on Thursday, but my friend Helena is here and we're ready. She's such a rock."

"That's wonderful to hear. And what else?"

"My hairdresser's made my hair look great – it had been thinning so much but this shorter, layered cut feels good."

"It suits you so well. And what else have you noticed?"

I wonder if she'll mention the book she was planning to read.

"When Helena got here at the weekend, we had a few of my other friends over and I cooked. It was so much fun."

"Oh wow. What did you make?"

"It was just a simple risotto with some prawns, crispy tofu, and bits and pieces like roasted broccoli. Everyone loved it and I really enjoyed being back in the kitchen."

"Sounds delicious and what was your day like yesterday?"

"Well, as it rained a little, we carried on the clearing which I started. I finished all the drawers before Helena arrived. But then she and I finished the wardrobe and the spare boxes and filled two huge bags full of things for the charity shop. Gone. Done."

"You've been busy..."

"Well, not only that, I weeded some of the garden after last week's session. And I read the whole book – not in one go – but a little reading every day has really suited me. In the afternoons and then a few pages before bed too."

"And how was the book?"

"It was so good. I'm going to get the other one she wrote. I've got to say it before you ask, I feel like an eight and a half today! It's only the operation that's stopping me hitting a nine or ten."

"Oh, that's brilliant. So, it sounds like you're noticing how the habit of doing small things you enjoy really helps you have more energy? And even if the operation feels daunting..."

"Yes... I think I'll book in to see you in three or four weeks, if that's okay? Just to get myself back on track faster once I'm through the pain killers and the time on the couch."

"Thank you, and I'll be happy to see you. Is there anything you'd like to focus on doing differently this week before you relax for this session?"

"Yes, I'll take Helena out for lunch – 12 noon tomorrow – to thank her for being here. There's no doubt her bubbly energy is helping me through this too."

"Well, that sounds like a plan to look forward to and well done for inviting her over and letting her know you needed help. Too many people struggle on without asking."

Judy smiles and lies back for a rest.

Judy

I step outside Deb's house and take in a peaceful, deep breath of the fresh air.

Well. What a sunny day again. Where shall I book for lunch tomorrow? What a beautiful front garden that house has... pretty flowers... and the sky is that brilliant blue... Time to get the bus back to Helena....

I start humming, as a familiar tune springs to mind, my limp slowing me down a little but not bothering me. As I go, I feel determined that the little voice inside my head will be as kind to me as I am to Emily. Always.

Debs Penrice: www.storyhealing.net

Unblocking your hidden stories:

What small changes might you make to improve your life?

When you look back on your life, what advice might your oldest, wisest self want to give you now?

15

HONOURING

Em Melrose

Stories help us capture the journey of life. They are powerful in how ordinary they can be and yet some are extraordinary too. They can be a way to honour relationships with others and mark shared moments in time together. When I met Em Melrose at the point when she was training to become a life celebrant, she reminded me of how letters also contain stories that can help us heal.

A letter of wishes to loved ones is an act of honouring, a place to guide and ground us when we feel lost in the depths of grief. Em says, "Every time I write a celebration of life service, I have the privilege of writing the story in honour of a life." At a time when grief can feel all consuming, storytelling can offer a place for healing, sharing stories of lives lived. Sometimes, a difficult part of losing someone is not knowing their last thoughts and wishes and carrying the heavy emotion of wondering if you've got it right. Em's fictionalised story shows us a journey of grief and profound connection through one such letter.

Peace of Mind

Sitting at one of their special places, she could feel the warmth of the sun on her back. Jock snuggled into her side, nudging her from time to time to remind her that he was there. His unconditional love was remarkable; he had a way of knowing that needed no explanation. She'd observed many trained therapy dogs in the past, and she knew that Jock was special. He was hers and how deeply blessed she was that he'd chosen her, long before what she was living through now. She was starting to understand the role that he came to play in her life. She drew him in close for, in that moment, she felt peace.

The warmth of a September evening was a time they had both cherished. She watched the clouds moving in the sky, the sounds of families enjoying themselves on the beach. She closed her eyes and tuned into the sounds of the waves, visualising the ebb and flow as the tide turned and started to come in.

She felt that familiar ball in her tummy again. She called it anger. He would never have wanted it to be this way. It had been there in the weeks before he passed and, on the days when she felt it rise up into her throat, she suppressed it. Nothing would bring him back to the place that he would want to be. He was free now and for that she was grateful, despite the loss she felt.

She knew the power of words, the hurt and pain that misplaced words could have on people, so she kept them inside, feeling their presence gnawing. Writing brought her some ease, better out than in, she thought, and at least it protected others from any unintentional hurt. Like many before him, he had gone too soon, so much life still to be lived, experiences to be shared, so much loving and laughing still to come.

Just like the ebb and flow of the tide, she felt her emotions come and go. She was learning to lean into them. Those emotions were more powerful some days than others, this grief thing was messy, unique. She had come to the place where it had no expiration date. She was the only person feeling her feelings and she knew, deep within, that he wouldn't want her to be stuck here for the rest of her life.

She brought her attention to her breath. She was starting to learn the power that it held to centre her when she focused on it. With each breath she could feel her body responding, releasing, calming her. Jock lent in closer, their breathing in sync. He felt it too.

She felt a subtle shift within herself, a sense of peace washed over her. She looked up to the sky and saw the sun's rays breaking through the clouds. In that moment, she felt the power of golden light upon her.

In the next breath, she was back in her thoughts. Life was cruel. She had faced situations that she would wish on no-one. Things that were beyond her control. Another breath, and she felt another shift, the movement of the clouds offering her a metaphor. Nothing remained still forever; her feelings and thoughts were just like the clouds moving through her mind. She had been drawn to come here today. Her afternoon client had cancelled, creating unexpected space. She knew she needed a change of scenery. She remembered getting into the car but couldn't remember driving here.

She brought her awareness to this thought. This was a place they had often come to together, to sit on the bench and look out at the shoreline. It brought them time and space. Neither felt the need to talk; there was a sense of deep connection between them.

She felt love wash over her, touching every part of her body. With each breath, she felt that love deeper within her. Tears started to flow, and she let them. She felt the release of the physical tension. Her tears held a cleansing power, and she felt connected with his essence for the first time. She felt the gentle breeze sweep over her, the movement in the clouds bringing the rays of the sun onto her face once again. She lifted her head and felt a bubble of laughter rise within her. The muscles in her face relaxed.

A sense of gratitude washed over her next. They had never spoken about his view on eternal life. What if this was his way of showing her? He knew her. What if today he was showing her that his essence is eternal?

She'd heard people talk about the signs from departed loved ones to show that they were still around – a favourite song on the radio, robins in the garden, a feather from nowhere, a familiar scent. As she tuned into these thoughts, she realised that these things had happened over the last few weeks. She smiled. He knew what he was doing. He was showing her patience. Maybe there was truth in the saying "the teacher will appear when the student is ready." She took a few deep breaths and smiled.

The day they found out that his diagnosis was incurable was the day she started to grieve, quietly and within. In truth, they had never spoken about his death or her life after. They channelled their energies into the present moment. His energy navigated the intensity of his treatment, while hers focused on keeping life as 'normal' as possible, with 'normal' constantly shifting as time progressed.

Years ago, when they wrote their wills, they had captured the critical bits. The children were young then, so guardianship mattered, and they'd included the obvious bits about funeral wishes. Beyond that, they'd only had occasional and impromptu conversations following the funerals of others – the good qualities of the person leading the service, the feelings they had been left with. Neither wrote anything down.

Jock nudged her out of her thoughts for a nano second. Feeling the cool air around her body, she pulled him close, the sun trapped in his silky fur bringing her warmth. The beach was quiet now. She wasn't ready to leave just yet. Jock was happy to be her warmth, and she felt the comfort of that.

Would things have been different if they had talked about his wishes and about hers too? Cancer doesn't care who it attaches to. What would be happening now if the shoe were on the other foot? One thing she knew for sure – he would be on top of the insurance renewals. Over the years, like many couples, they had each fallen into roles within their marriage. How could we have become so complacent, she asked herself.

Her thoughts now moved to the present. Some might say she was mad to move house so quickly after he'd gone. Ironically, this was one of the things they had talked about and had started to plan together, living for the moment, all of them together. Call it synchronicity, but only days after he passed, she found a house that met all their needs. It was the children who saw the sign. It couldn't have been more obvious and it was the affirmation she needed. They say that moving house is one of the most stressful things we do. Add losing a loved one to that mix... well, I'm sure many people thought she was mad. But that's the thing, grief has no pattern or path, it is unique to all of us. For her, it kept the family moving forward.

A sensitivity washed over her. There had been moments when she felt judged for the decisions she was making. It was less what people said and more what they didn't say. The feelings were hers to process. No one else was walking in her shoes, along her unique life path, and she wasn't walking in theirs. She was learning to release these feelings of judgement and, instead, appreciate those around her for caring and loving her in their own way. She was learning so much about herself.

Jock nudged her again and she smiled to herself. It must be getting close to his dinner time. By now, the sun was starting to set. They had loved to come here at this time of day, an unspoken knowing that, as the sun sets today, it will rise again tomorrow; yet, for us human beings, there is no promise of tomorrow.

Jock was getting restless, ready to move on. Being here today had enabled an unexpected layer of release and healing. She smiled and took some deep breaths, the fresh sea air filling her lungs with an energy that felt familiar, energising, hopeful. She looked up to the sky and felt loving tears fill her eyes. Thank you, my darling, she whispered.

She slept deeply and wholesomely, better than she had in months. Getting out of bed, she drew back the curtains and opened the window, welcoming the new day in and the birdsong with it. The chorus was somehow richer, more vibrant, today.

He had the superpower of asking questions, of unlocking access to the answers that people held within, tucked safely beneath years of automatic responses. He'd asked questions of her yesterday, even though he wasn't physically present. He had left her with the most precious gift of giving herself the time and space to get curious about her thoughts and feelings in a place where she felt safe and connected.

She walked downstairs and into the kitchen, the comforting sensation of the carpet pile beneath her feet transforming with the change in temperature as she stepped onto the cold kitchen tiles. As she waited for the kettle to boil, she looked out the window.

There he was, Mr Robin on the fence. He seemed to stay longer than usual and it seemed to her that their eyes locked in a moment of recognition and connection.

She knew what her purpose was for today.

Taking her cup of hot tea, she sat at her laptop, wrapping her hands around the warm cup. She planted her feet firmly on the floor and took some deep breaths. Today she was going to write her letter of wishes.

She knew it would be challenging, yet it would honour the peace of mind she wanted to create for the children. It would be a priceless gift and she would channel any discomfort she felt into her love for them. She reflected back on yesterday's sunset, and her thought that no one's tomorrow is promised. She was still navigating this new chapter, and she knew there was no manual for grief. But what she could leave them was guidance on the practical things, suggestions about how she'd like to be laid to rest; things that, in moments of wobble, might be an anchor for them.

She knew that, in this act of love, she was making a commitment to herself and to them to revisit this letter. She had no intention of dying and she released the nagging thought that 'by talking or writing about it would attract it.' Instead, this was an act of love that someday, when her sun did not rise, an eternal golden thread of connection would bring them some measure of comfort and guidance.

Before she began, she made a few commitments to herself: her words would flow as if she were speaking to them; if she needed to stop today, she would; whatever guidance she gave them would be more than they had right now. This evening, when they came together for their weekly family dinner, she would share her experience of the past twenty-four hours. If they wanted to talk, she would hold space for them to do so. She trusted that her own golden thread of connection to loved ones who had passed would guide her.

When she finally departed, many years later, this was the letter she left for them:

My loves,

You are reading this because I am no longer here. My letter of wishes has evolved over the years from that very first conversation we had. You were not ready to talk about life without me, but as time has passed, I have gently sowed seeds. I feel you will be surprised by how much you already know. This letter will be a point of reference, a place to steady you, and my hope is to give you direction when you feel lost. I never imagined that the experience of writing my own letter of wishes would become a way for me to help others to create peace of mind for their loved ones too. Writing this letter, and all that followed, was a saving grace that helped me to channel my losses in a healthier way. On so many occasions, I have had the privilege of holding space for those in the early days of grief to celebrate their loved ones. So, my first reminder to you is, in every situation, you will find something to help you learn and grow. And I am forever grateful for the support you have shown me, as I rehearse the services to honour those souls that have passed. Ironic as it has often felt, being able to channel my energy to support others has allowed a deeper layer of healing to take place within me; healing from wounds that I unknowingly carried into my adult life, and from beliefs that weren't serving me. When I chose to accept that I would always be 'a work in progress human being,' life began to flow with ease, even in choppy waters.

I know, what you're thinking: Mum, get on with it!

I trust that this helps and guides you as you navigate the next chapter of your lives.

While this is never going to be a manual for 'life after me,' in the same way that I sometimes wished for a manual to know how to be a mum, my hope is that it will offer you support and a place to remember that you are never alone. I am only ever a thought away. Trust in your inner wisdom. You hold the answers here. Be patient and kind to yourselves. I know that your hearts are hurting. We never shied away from the conversation about death and that it would come to us all one day. But the truth is that, when you are feeling loss to your core, grief hurts so deeply, accept that this is all part of the circle of life.

I am so proud of the adults that you have become. Trust in your inner strength and believe that I am always around you. There is a golden thread of light that connects us, as it did from the day that your dad went, and you trusted that. (Remember the day you found our new home?) It is no different with me. You'll know and believe it's true. Our love is eternal, and I am deeply blessed that I was part of your lives for so long, to watch you grow into the beautiful human beings that you are. I am grateful for the lessons that you taught me about loving unconditionally. I was always working to improve my patience! I see how you engage with your own families, the values that you continue to honour from your own childhoods and how those values will continue to live on as your children nurture their own families in time.

We've talked in the past about how I wanted to celebrate my life. But the truth is, that you might be feeling a bit different now that I am gone. I have captured my thoughts and wishes here. I respect that my service will be a place for you to come in support of each other. My essence will be around you, but my physical presence will not. So, what I am saying, in my wordy way, is if you feel you want to do something else, that's OK.

I ask that you celebrate me. I have been blessed with so many wonderful experiences in this life, even the toughest times have brought learning. I hope that I leave this earth with people remembering me as 'a good human being' for that was what I set out to be every day. I would love to know that you are surrounded by love and support as you lay my body to rest. As you know, there is a legal process to 'dispose of my body' (it sounds kinder when we say 'lay to rest'); so, as per my will, which you do need to adhere to, my request is that I am cremated. If you choose a direct cremation for me, I want it to be a local one.

I encourage you to come together to bring some physical closure. How you choose to do this is up to you. In my experiences with other families, closure is a significant element of the healing journey, so do what feels right. If you decide on a direct cremation, there's no rush to hold a memorial celebration – it's my physical presence that has gone. There will be lots of practical things that will need your energy in the early days, and I hope that, with this letter, I have eased things a little for you with practical information. Talking about a coffin was always too raw. Just keep it simple, the funeral director will guide you. If you decide to have a service, here are some things that I'd like you to consider. I was never blessed with a great voice, but God loves a trier, right?

So, I would like "This little light of mine" to be sung. It can be belted out and you can't sing it without smiling! For readings and poems, there are so many that I have spoken and recorded over the years, but Donna Ashworth will always be a favourite of mine. Flowers. They must be sunflowers. Don't go mad with them if you are having a service, but please plant seeds every year. If they don't grow, you'll learn how to do it better the following year. I'll save you the faff of finding natural fibre clothes to dress me in. If you can, choose a coloured gown for me, preferably bright pink!

As for my ashes, I want you to decide. For years, I shared with you that I hold the belief that my essence lives on with you forever. If you want some ideas, I love that we can send our ashes into space (you know how I always said that we are all connected universally, so that would be pretty cool). My happy places? Well, you know where these are, so maybe scatter me in a few of them. If you choose to use my ashes to make something and that brings you comfort, then I am happy that you're happy, and there's no rush.

Now, on to more practical things. I want to make it as simple as possible for you to deal with my estate. I can't promise that I've covered everything, but I hope that this makes the journey a little easier to navigate. We've spoken in the past about things that I wanted each of you to have and that's all documented in my will. But I know that one of the traits you love about me is my sentimentality! Yes, it's years now since I emptied your grandparents' home. For years after, I carried some guilt and fear about letting go of things that I knew had really mattered to them. Do you remember that I held on to seven bibles because I didn't know which one was the family one. We got there in the end, didn't we!

I don't want that for you. So, over the years, I have subtly marked things that I hope you will keep in our family. It will be like another game of hunt the thimble for you! If you aren't ready to let things go, put them into storage. Take your time. I know that some of my things are of no interest to you. I respect that. But rather than taking them to the charity shop or amenity site, I have left you a separate list of contact names to help and guide you.

There's no getting away from the fact that it's going to take some time to work through my personal administration. I am so glad that I invested in the services of a financial advisor many years ago. They will be able to take the lead in contacting the organisations that I have invested with, but there are others that only you can deal with. I have kept a list of all the key services that I use in a digital vault. You'll find the access code to that vault in the attached letter. This is going to make life much easier for you. I am so glad that I got into the habit of updating it, as I knew it would always be there for you when you needed it. I'm sure you'll be thanking me many times over!

You will need more copies of my death certificate than you think, so get a few copies. You will need these to be able to process my estate without much delay. The funeral will be a time and place to say goodbye and start to process the next chapter in your lives. Grief is the weirdest of things. I remember once hearing it described as the place that love has nowhere to go. Those days when you want to pick up the phone and tell me your news will knock you over. So will anniversaries and birthdays and other days that were special only to us.

We've talked over the years about our grief. There is no right or wrong way, only your way. All I ask is that you remember to be kind to yourselves on the days that feel the hardest and to be kind and patient with each other. I am no longer physically there with you, but my essence is always around you. Look for the signs that remind you of this and never doubt their truth, for I am always only ever a thought away. To have shared my life with you has been an honour. You have taught me so much. Every time I have revisited this letter, life has brought us new challenges and experiences to cherish as, every day, with open hearts, we learn how to be good human beings.

My sunrise will not come again, but trust that our eternal love is forever.

Mum, Kate. x x x

Em Melrose: www.yourcelebrant.life

UNBLOCKING YOUR HIDDEN STORIES:

What legacy would you like to leave?

How would you like your loved ones to honour your wishes?

ACKNOWLEDGEMENTS

Shortly after I started writing the original version of 'Stories that Heal', I was walking in the park with my dear friend Lesley, saying how stuck I'd got and how much admiration I have for anyone who writes a whole book. Enormous thanks go to her, because she reminded me that listening to others' stories was my core focus as therapist. So, it was a great idea to gather my co-authors and hear their stories. This book would not have happened without that spark of an idea to use case studies and short stories to highlight how significant stories are to us all. It's been said before and no doubt I will say it again: stories heal, and stories inspire.

Sharing stories with my brilliant friends tops up my energy and I'm grateful for all of you; especially you Nigel, and Duncan, because I treasure our chats to keep me inspired, thank you. And Angus Penrice, you are simply the most patient sounding board, which I appreciate from the bottom of my heart. There's one person I wish you had met – who I knew as Gramma – she was formally known as Joan (Ellen) Esworthy. This book is dedicated to her and our family. Yet since she's been gone, we've extended our family with our two awesome daughters, who make life so much fun – thank you girls.

Along my business journey, I've joined a wonderful tribe led by amazing coaches, Wendy Ismail, Adam and Becca Brooks, and created circles of my own. I launched my first book writing group with Helen Hart and I'm hugely grateful that my work with her authors led me to hosting masterclasses to encourage more people to enjoy writing. One of those authors is Richard Sutcliffe, whose wise yet humorous counsel helped me bring this book to life. Helen also introduced me to our editor, Martina Tyrell, whose support was invaluable in refining and bringing our stories together. All the while, Abigail Barnes has played a high-energy role in supporting me as I developed the concept, and found our talented designer – thank you.

On that note of writing more, I'd like to thank all of my co-authors again for taking the leap to write and publish your stories with mine. It will be an honour to see you write your next books or share your stories in other ways in the future.

For our readers, thank you for taking the time to read this book and you're welcome to contact me or any of the co-authors via their web links if you'd like more information or some help to share your story. I'd love to stay in touch and hear which stories you resonated with the most and answer any questions you have. Drop me an email or message me:

Email: debra@storyhealing.net
Instagram: @storyhealingwithdebra
LinkedIn: www.linkedin.com/in/debrapenrice27/
Facebook: @storyhealingwithdebra
Website: www.storyhealing.net

Best wishes and happy writing, Debs

About Debs Penrice

www.storyhealing.net

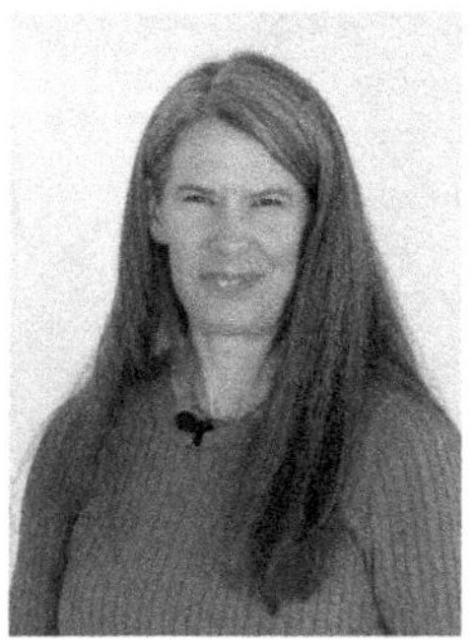

Debs is the founder of Story Healing, where she blends solution-focused therapy and writing coaching. Her career evolved from storytelling in marketing and business, writing client success stories for businesses to listen to their client's feedback and build trust beyond testimonials. Working for a hybrid publisher, SilverWood Books, she launched an online writing group. Today, she supports men and women to release emotional and psychological blocks, and overcome anxiety. She helps clients change their inner stories and enjoy life more. She practises meditation, Reiki, singing and swimming to balance her creativity and energy. She lives in Bristol with her Scottish husband and their two lively teenage daughters. Visit her website via the QR code:

About Abigail Barnes

www.abigailbarnes.com

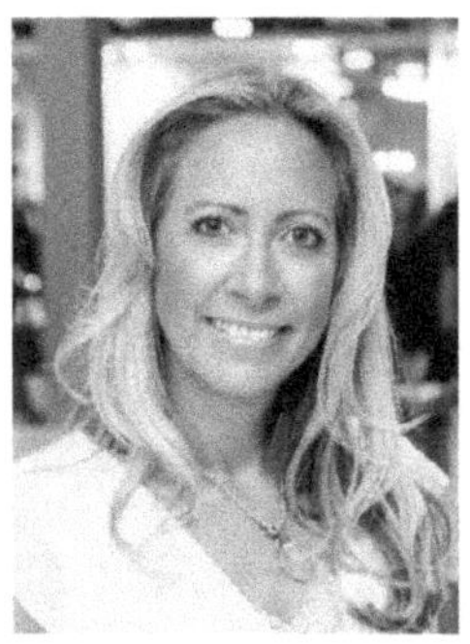

Abigail Barnes is the founder and CEO of Success by Design Training. She is an award-winning entrepreneur, author, international speaker, marketing strategist, and transformational coach. She is the creator of the Idea to Author framework and the globally recognised 888 Formula, powerful tools designed to help individuals turn their ideas into books and maximise the time they have to create the life they want. She is the host of The Time Management Podcast, where she shares practical strategies and inspiring stories from her own journey, alongside insights from special guests. Visit her website via the QR code:

About Alison Westlake

www.thehealingpath.uk

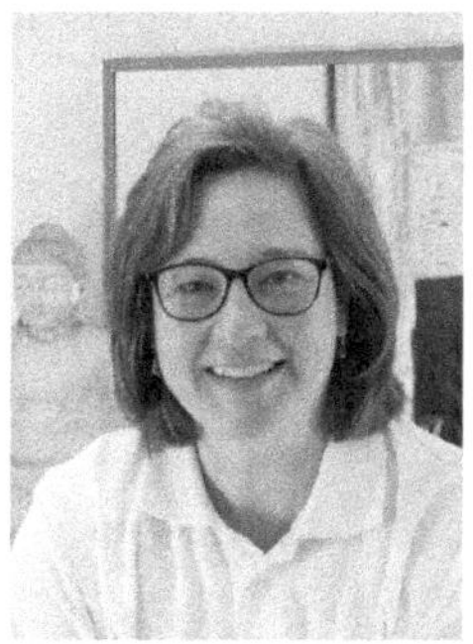

Alison is a holistic massage therapist and therapeutic coach, assisting people who are experiencing mental, emotional and physical challenges. Her work is person centred, tailoring sessions to meet her clients' needs. Alison's approach is intuitive, caring, reflective and explorative. Her journey as a therapist began when she suffered a herniated disc. Through the use of essential oils, massage, reflexology, exercise and a positive mindset, she was able to heal and avoid surgery. Alison's career in holistic massage followed supporting students with autism. Alison lives with her husband, and has a daughter, a son and family dog in Bristol. She enjoys many forms of dancing, cooking and Tai chi. Daily exercise, meditation, and mindset work are integral parts of her life. Visit her website via the QR code:

ABOUT ANGIE HAYES

www.angie-hayes-hypnotherapy.co.uk

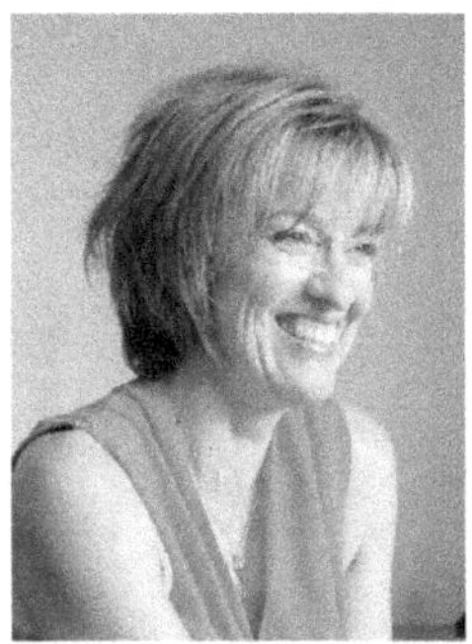

Angie is a therapist near the coast in North Somerset, working with clients using an integrative approach that combines hypnosis and solution-focused brief therapy. She is a mentor and continuous professional development trainer for newly qualified therapists. After starting out in accountancy and spending much of her career in banking and finance, she found her true calling in helping people navigate change, through stories, insight and healing. Angie is passionate about helping others understand themselves more deeply. She believes that when we take the time to reflect, we open doors to transformation and growth. Outside of work, Angie is a proud petrolhead who loves cars, motorbikes, long walks and the company of animals. Visit her website via the QR code:

About Becky Clark

www.beckyclarkcoaching.com

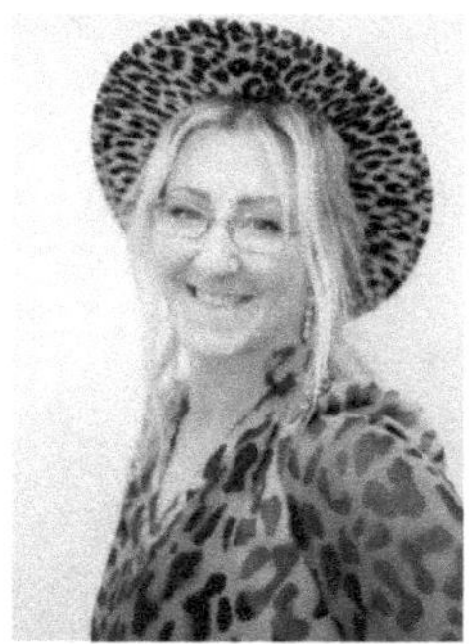

Becky runs several thriving ventures, from podiatry and foot health clinics to Goldney House, a holistic wellness and business centre. Her work reflects her belief in whole-person transformation and somatic self-awareness. Becky helps people attune to their nervous systems to expand, lead with ease, and create success without self-abandonment. She created the FLIP Formula™, her trademark nervous system reset to catch spirals before they turn into anxiety or overwhelm, which is grounded in shaking, pulsing and bioenergetics. She is also trained in TRE® (Tension & Trauma Releasing Exercises), which recalibrate the nervous system. When she's not running businesses, Becky is a devoted mum to her little one and occasionally sneaks in time to play the drums. Visit her website via the QR code:

ABOUT CAROLINE SMITH MCLEAN

www.carolinesmithmcleanhypnotherapy.com

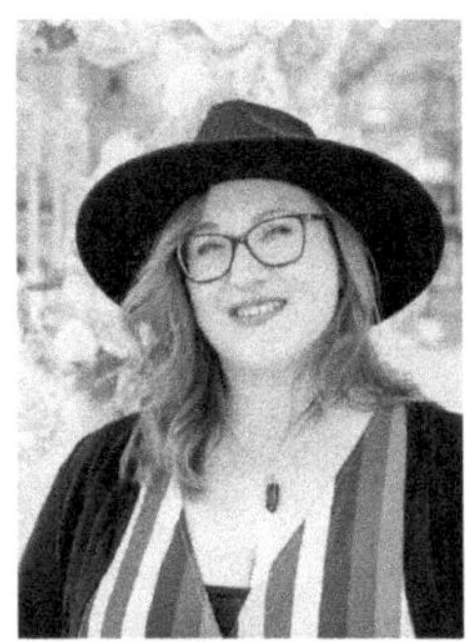

Caroline is a hypnotherapist, timeline therapist and breathwork facilitator who helps women attract love and success by clearing patterns and blind spots that hold them back. Her work is all about deep, lasting shifts that feel aligned and empowering. She came to this work through her own healing journey in relationships and business and her lived experience shaped her calm, intuitive and, sometimes, lovingly blunt approach. Her work isn't about quick fixes or perfection, it's about helping women come home to themselves, trust what they feel, and create a life that genuinely fits. Outside of sessions, Caroline is mum to two brilliant teenage boys, a fan of wild swimming, and is happiest wandering on long walks or van-tripping in what she affectionately calls her "bed on wheels." Visit her website via the QR code:

About Chris Stanley

www.thesoulalignmentacademy.com

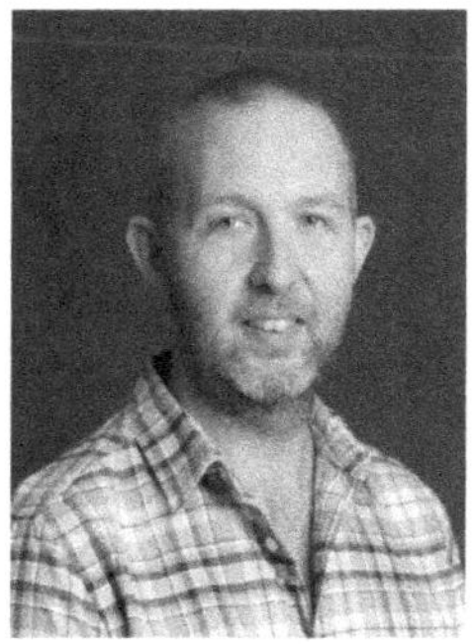

Chris Stanley is a spiritual development mentor, intuitive coach and founder of The Soul Alignment Academy. He supports individuals on their path of reconnection, helping them deepen their intuitive gifts, heal limiting patterns and rediscover who they truly are beneath layers of expectation and noise. Chris shares meditations and leads weekly development circles and one-to-one sessions that blend psychic and mediumship training with personal empowerment and soul remembrance. Chris is the author of 'You are already psychic'. and 'Discover Your Spirit Guides', offering practical guidance into connecting with your spiritual skills and team. Based in the Forest of Dean, Chris also offers forest therapy. Visit his website via the QR code:

About Em Melrose

www.yourcelebrant.life

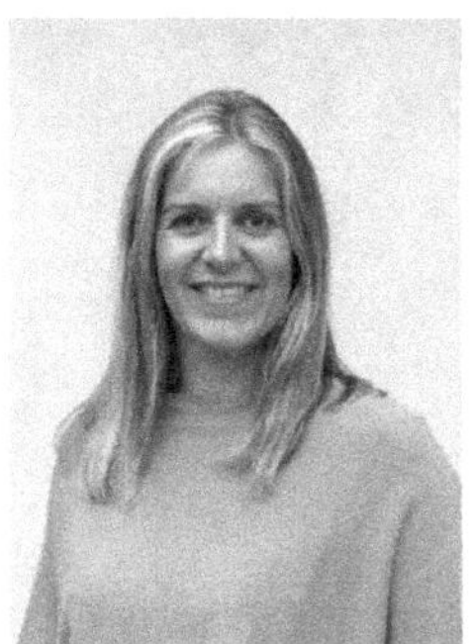

Em Melrose is a leadership coach and Reiki master, whose life was transformed by deep personal loss, when she lost both parents in 2019 and her husband in 2021. Em walks purposefully with her grief, supporting others to heal on their journeys. She is an Independent Celebrant, offering heartfelt support to individuals and families as they honour life in Celebration of Life and Memorial Services. Em creates compassionate space for people to reflect and begin to heal. She encourages open conversations about legacy and gently advocates for creating a letter of wishes, offering peace of mind and clarity. Em lives in West Wales, has two daughters and a very special dog. She is living this chapter of her life with more courage because "Nobody's tomorrow is promised." Visit her website via the QR code:

About Gerwyn Tumelty

www.coronprojects.co.uk

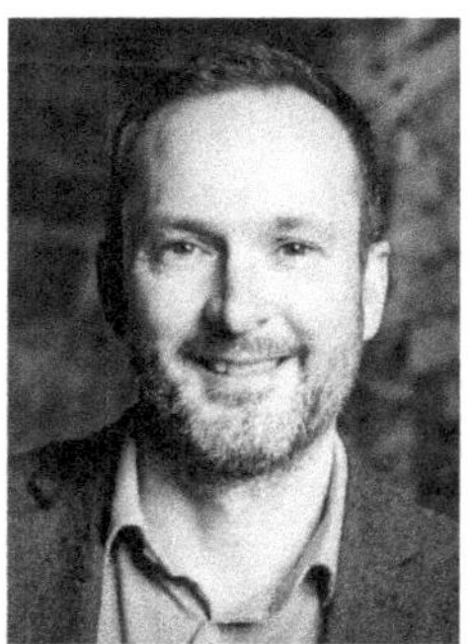

Gerwyn is founder of Coron Projects, supporting project managers in engineering and construction to lead with clarity, purpose and self-awareness. He believes project delivery is more than process and profit, it's about people. He champions a reflective approach to leadership, especially where pressure, performance and pace can take priority over wellbeing. A husband with three sons, Gerwyn lives in Pontarddulais near Swansea. His youngest has additional learning needs, which along with his experiences of chronic pain, neurosurgery and significant mental struggles, has profoundly shaped his outlook. These personal challenges were a catalyst for change, forcing him to re-evaluate how he worked and lived. Visit his website via the QR code:

About Kimberley Vallis

www.theedventureproject.co.uk

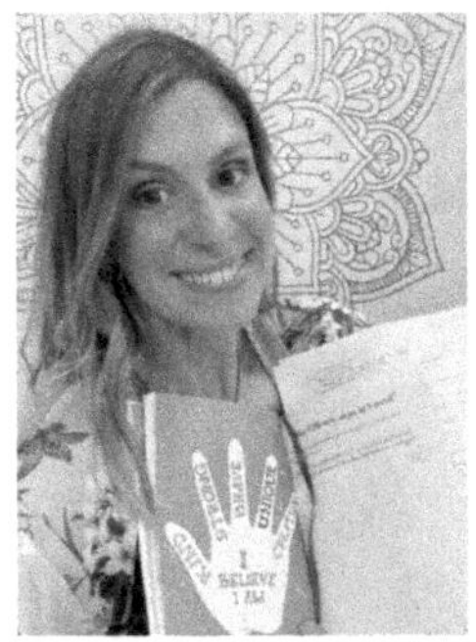

Kimberley Vallis is an alternative educator, intuitive wellness mentor and founder of The Edventure Project CiC, and Serendipity with Kimberley. Both are nature-based community-rooted initiatives offering purpose-led empowerment that supports children and adults to thrive, grow and listen outside of conventional systems. With a background in mainstream teaching and a passion for alternative education, Kimberley blends her experience of holistic wellness practices, such as Reiki and sound healing, with her zest for mentoring to help others to reconnect with their values, rhythms and true selves. She finds solace and energy from the support of her own family, her incredible husband Tony, her three sons and her stepson. Visit her website via the QR code:

About Lisa Williams Edgar

www.newhorizontraining.co.uk

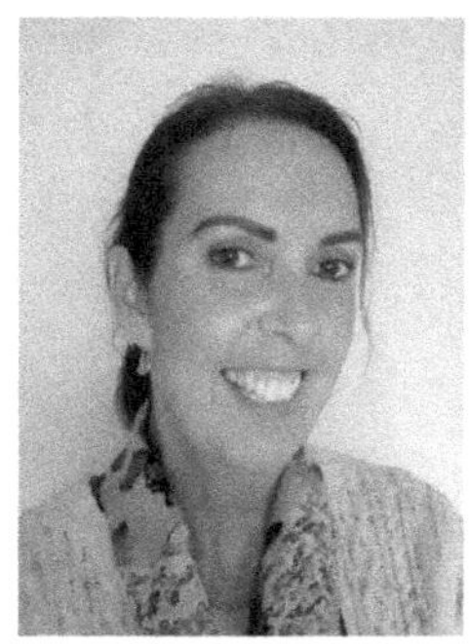

Lisa is a clinical integrative hypnotherapist with training in psychotherapy, cognitive behavioural therapy, and NLP. As founder of New Horizon Training and senior lecturer with Ayurva Academy, she is a senior lecturer, co-writing and delivering training and continuous professional development workshops. She is a supervisor for other therapists to support them to grow their confidence and skills. Her work was recognised with two awards for Most Trusted Clinical Hypnotherapist in North Somerset. Her journey as a therapist followed a career in financial services, after her personal life-changing experience with hypnotherapy. Based in a quiet village in Somerset, Lisa's work reflects her belief in new beginnings and the power of purposeful change. Visit her website via the QR code:

About Richard Sutcliffe

www.findingmaccouk.wordpress.com

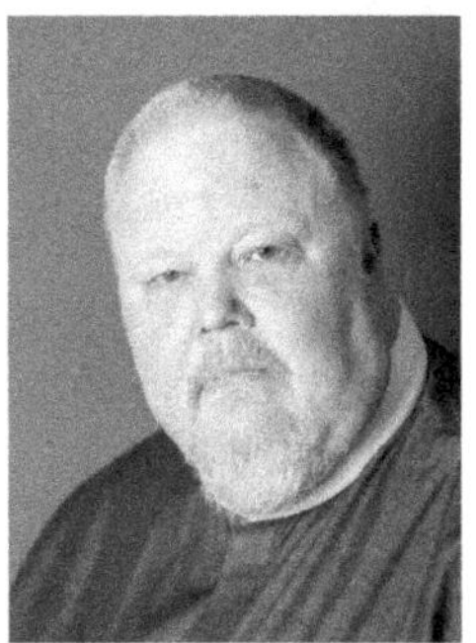

Reverend Richard Sutcliffe lives in a village in Hampshire where he is a part-time Church of England priest, working as part of a wider local ministry team. This gives him time with his sister, nephews and their growing families, his dogs, and to indulge in his interest in art. As a qualified accountant, he worked in London as a financial regulator, then retired early to enjoy the countryside with his family and dogs. Richard wrote his first book, *Finding Mac*, to help the memories of his son to live on. Richard and his late wife Swee welcomed eight-year-old Mac into their lives, navigating the highs and lows of adoption. But Mac was killed on his motorbike after his sixteenth birthday, and though overwhelmingly positive, *Finding Mac* deals honestly with the feelings of parents facing the death of their child, available via the QR code:

About Tor Obermaier

www.tor-obermaier.live.baluu.io

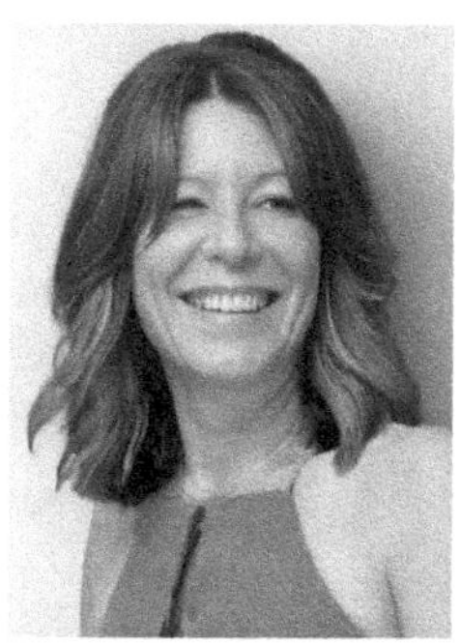

Tor is a Nia dance teacher, personal development coach and massage therapist, helping people feel more present and at ease in their bodies. Her professional journey began as a primary school teacher before moving into senior management in schools for children with special needs, supporting hard-to-reach teenagers. Although she loved her work, Tor felt called to explore new ways of facilitating personal growth. She is inspired by the power of Nia, movement and music to heal, connect and transform. Her curiosity remains boundless, with Qi Gong as her next adventure in mind-body practice. Tor lives on the border of the Wye Valley and the Forest of Dean with her husband, and is a proud mother to three daughters, and a grandmother. She also enjoys singing, acting and exploring historical sites. Visit her website via the QR code:

UNTOLD

AND

RETOLD

Coming soon

Would you like to take part in the next volume of Stories that Heal?
We will be launching the programme with the opportunity for
therapists, coaches, and people who'd like to start their writing
journey with fiction. You'll be welcome to work with Debs on
releasing any subconscious blocks before you start writing.

For a free download on 3 steps to release your blocks and raise your
energy levels, visit storyhealing.net

Contact Debs Penrice for more information.

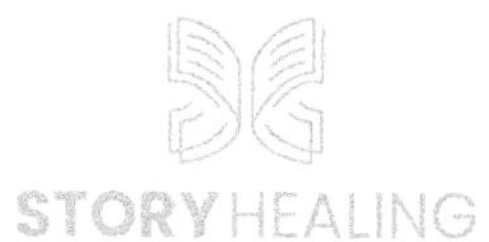

www.ingramcontent.com/pod-product-compliance
Lightning Source LLC
Chambersburg PA
CBHW051515030726
47592CB00006B/2268